When Disaster Strikes

Second Edition

OPUS COMMUNICATIONS
A Division of hcPro

When Disaster Strikes, Second Edition is published by Opus Communications, Inc., a subsidiary of HCPro Corp.

Copyright 2002 Opus Communications, Inc., a subsidiary of HCPro Corp.

All rights reserved. Printed in the United States of America. 5 4 3 2 1

ISBN 1-57839-178-4

No part of this publication may be reproduced, in any form or by any means, without prior written consent of Opus Communications or the Copyright Clearance Center (978/750-8400). Please notify us immediately if you have received an unauthorized copy.

Opus Communications provides information resources for the healthcare industry.

Neither HCPro Corp. nor Opus Communications, Inc., is affiliated in any way with the Joint Commission on Accreditation of Healthcare Organizations.

Kimberly Raines, Managing Editor
Scott Wallask, Contributing Editor
Jean St. Pierre, Creative Director
Mike Mirabello, Senior Graphic Artist
Shane Katz, Cover Designer
Suzanne Perney, Publisher

Advice given is general. Readers should consult professional counsel for specific legal, ethical, or clinical questions.

Arrangements can be made for quantity discounts.

For more information, contact:

Opus Communications
P.O. Box 1168
Marblehead, MA 01945
Telephone: 800/650-6787 or 781/639-1872
Fax: 781/639-2982
E-mail: customer_service@hcpro.com

Visit Opus Communications at its World Wide Web sites:
***www.hcmarketplace.com*, *www.hcpro.com*, and *www.himinfo.com*.**

Table of Contents

Introduction

The world changed on September 11, 2001. The unthinkable became a reality following the devastating terrorist attacks on New York City and Washington, DC. These events sparked a new era of awareness for healthcare organizations, and a need for more information. That's why we've created this updated version of "When Disaster Strikes." In this second edition, you'll find case studies on lessons learned by healthcare organizations following the attacks on the World Trade Center and the Pentagon.

Defining disaster

The Joint Commission on Accreditation of Healthcare Organizations (JCAHO) defines a disaster as a man-made or natural event that significantly disrupts the environment of care, such as damage to the organization's building(s) and grounds due to severe wind storms, tornadoes, earthquakes, or hurricanes. A disaster can also be an event that disrupts care and treatment of patients, such as loss of utilities (water, power, telephones) due to floods, civil disturbances (riots, shootings, massacres), terrorism, traffic accidents, fires, or other emergencies within the organization or in the surrounding community. The results of these disasters can vary from widespread infection to utility failure to loss of needed medical supplies.

Is your facility ready?

Your first step against disasters should be taken long before the actual event occurs. Although there is nothing you can do to prevent a disaster, you can take precautions to protect yourself and the organization's residents from its effects.

The key is to develop an effective emergency preparedness plan (also known as a disaster plan) and to establish an incident command system (ICS). The emergency preparedness plan should be a comprehensive, systematic, and easy-to-follow strategy for dealing with disasters. An ICS should serve as a hierarchy of responsibilities for the disaster plan and be based on simple organizational concepts.

There are a few important guidelines to remember when developing these strategies. First, no matter how complex an operation is, there are distinct groups within it that have responsibility for specific functions. Next, keep in mind that one individual can successfully manage only five to seven people. Finally, remember that, without clear methods and lines of communication, even the best plans cannot be carried out. (For a sample emergency preparedness management plan and ICS, please see Appendix B.)

How will this book help?

Although it is not something that we like to think about, the fact is that every facility is vulnerable to disasters. Would your facility be prepared to react quickly and effectively? What would be your first move?

It is important to remember that different healthcare facilities deal with disasters in different ways. This book will give you a look into the real-life experiences of various hospitals around the country and how they dealt with man-made and natural disasters. What did they do right? What did they do wrong? How could they have been better prepared? The appendices also provide tools, checklists, and valuable information to help better prepare your facility for when disaster strikes.

Chapter One

Bioterrorism

Anthrax: Frequently asked questions

The following is a list of frequently asked questions about anthrax. These come from the Division of Bacterial and Mycotic Diseases, part of the Centers for Disease Control and Prevention's (CDC) National Center for Infectious Diseases.

What is anthrax?

Anthrax is an acute infectious disease caused by the spore-forming bacterium Bacillus anthracis. Anthrax most commonly occurs in wild and domestic lower vertebrates (cattle, sheep, goats, camels, antelopes, and other herbivores), but it can also occur in humans when they are exposed to infected animals or tissue from infected animals.

Why has anthrax become a current issue?

Because anthrax is considered to be a potential agent for use in biological warfare, the Department of Defense has begun mandatory vaccination of all active duty military personnel who might be involved in conflict.

How common is anthrax, and who can get it?

Anthrax is most common in agricultural regions, where it occurs in animals. These regions include South and Central America, Southern and Eastern Europe, Asia, Africa, the Caribbean, and the Middle East. When anthrax affects humans, it is usually due to an occupational exposure to infected animals or their products. Workers who are exposed to dead animals and animal products from other countries where anthrax is more common may become infected with B. anthracis (industrial anthrax). Anthrax in wild livestock has occurred in the United States.

How is anthrax transmitted?

Anthrax infection can occur in three forms: cutaneous (skin), inhalation, and gastrointestinal. B. anthracis spores can live in the soil for many years, and humans can become infected with anthrax by handling products from infected animals or by inhaling anthrax spores from contaminated animal products. Anthrax can also be spread by eating undercooked meat from infected animals. It is rare to find infected animals in the United States.

What are the symptoms of anthrax?

Symptoms of the disease vary depending on how the disease was contracted, but symptoms usually occur within seven days.

Cutaneous: Most (about 95%) anthrax infections occur when the bacterium enters a cut or abrasion on the skin, such as when handling contaminated wool, hides, leather, or hair products (especially goat hair) of infected animals. Skin infection begins as a raised, itchy bump that resembles an insect bite, but within one or two days, it develops into a vesicle and then a painless ulcer, usually 1 - 3 cm in diameter, with a characteristic black necrotic (dying) area in the center. Lymph glands in the adjacent area may swell. About 20% of untreated cases of cutaneous anthrax will result in death. Deaths are rare with appropriate antimicrobial therapy.

Inhalation: Initial symptoms may resemble a common cold. After several days, the symptoms may progress to severe breathing problems and shock. Inhalation anthrax is usually fatal.

Intestinal: The intestinal disease form of anthrax may follow the consumption of contaminated meat and is characterized by an acute inflammation of the intestinal tract. Initial signs of nausea, loss of appetite, vomiting, and fever is followed by abdominal pain, vomiting of blood, and severe diarrhea. Intestinal anthrax results in death in 25% to 60% of cases.

Where is anthrax usually found?

Anthrax can be found globally. It is more common in developing countries or countries without veterinary public health programs. Certain regions of the world (South and Central America, Southern and Eastern Europe, Asia, Africa, the Caribbean, and the Middle East) report more anthrax in animals than others.

Can anthrax be spread from person to person?

Direct, person-to-person spread of anthrax is extremely unlikely to occur. Communicability is not a concern in managing or visiting with patients with inhalation anthrax.

Is there a way to prevent infection?

In countries where anthrax is common and vaccination levels of animal herds are low, humans should avoid contact with livestock and animal products, and avoid eating meat that has not been properly slaughtered and cooked. Also, an anthrax vaccine has been licensed for use in humans. The vaccine is reported to be 93% effective in protecting against anthrax.

What is the anthrax vaccine?

The anthrax vaccine is manufactured and distributed by BioPort

Corporation, Lansing, MI. The vaccine is a cell-free filtrate vaccine, which means it contains no dead or live bacteria in the preparation. The final product contains no more than 2.4 mg of aluminum hydroxide as adjuvant. Anthrax vaccines intended for animals should not be used in humans.

Who should get vaccinated against anthrax?

The Advisory Committee on Immunization Practices has recommend anthrax vaccination for the following groups:

- Persons who work directly with the organism in the laboratory.
- Persons who work with imported animal hides or furs in areas where standards are insufficient to prevent exposure to anthrax spores.
- Persons who handle potentially infected animal products in high-incidence areas. (The incidence is low in the United States, but veterinarians who travel to work in other countries where the incidence is higher should consider being vaccinated.)
- Military personnel deployed to areas with a high risk for exposure to the organism (as when it is used as a biological warfare weapon).

The anthrax Vaccine Immunization Program in the U.S. Army Surgeon General's Office can be reached at 1-877-GETVACC (1-877-438-8222) or at *www.anthrax.osd.mil.*

Pregnant women should be vaccinated only if absolutely necessary.

What is the protocol for anthrax vaccination?

The immunization consists of three subcutaneous injections given two weeks apart, followed by three additional subcutaneous injections given at six, 12, and 18 months. Annual booster injections of the vaccine are recommended thereafter.

Are there adverse reactions to the anthrax vaccine?

Mild local reactions occur in 30% of recipients and consist of slight tenderness and redness at the injection site. Severe local reactions are infrequent and consist of extensive swelling of the forearm in addition to the local reaction. Systemic reactions occur in less than 0.2% of recipients.

How is anthrax diagnosed?

Anthrax is diagnosed by isolating B. anthracis from the blood, skin lesions, or respiratory secretions or by measuring specific antibodies in the blood of persons with suspected cases.

Is there a treatment for anthrax?

Doctors can prescribe effective antibiotics. To be effective, treatment should be initiated early. If left untreated, the disease can be fatal.

Where can I get more information about the recent decision that requires the armed services to be vaccinated?

The Department of Defense recommends that servicemen and -women contact their chain of command about questions concerning the vaccine and its distribution. The anthrax Vaccine Immunization Program in the U.S. Army Surgeon General's Office can be reached at 1-877-GETVACC (1-877-438-8222) or at *www.anthrax.osd.mil.*

Source: CDC

Communication is key in attack response

In any bioterrorist or chemical attack, the scale of the incident will create a demand for public information. In most cases, at least some of the information will not be readily available while the incident develops. Absent clear and credible information, speculation may reign and increase the stress and pressure resulting from the incident, especially on the hospital and its staff. Planned and structured arrangements for communication throughout the incident and during its response are critical components of hospital and community preparedness.

Internal communications

Single channel network

Hospitals need an ongoing, open channel of communication with emergency response teams that may have first contact with the incident scene. In a mass casualty incident, don't limit the channel of communications so that the Emergency Medical Service (EMS) unit has to use a different channel or means of contact with each organization. Use a community-wide network on the same channel. Test the network daily, with the test rotating across the various healthcare facilities and EMS shifts. Build redundant backup capability into the preparedness plan in case the usual means of communications fail. The backup capability also requires regular testing.

Relatives of the victims

The arrival of casualties will be accompanied by calls from family and friends seeking to learn the person's whereabouts and condition. These well-meaning calls can rapidly overload the hospital's telephone system and isolate the facility. Community-wide mass casualty preparedness plans will improve the responsiveness of healthcare organizations if they include a single, community site for obtaining patient locator information. In many communities, the Red Cross is equipped to serve, and experienced in serving, as this third-party, off-site source of information.

External communication

A bioterrorist event can become even more disastrous if every organization in the community attempts to establish its own media briefings. Unaware of what others are saying, and, despite the best of intentions, the use of different words and phrases can confuse the public and undermine the trust essential to the "orderly chaos" of a well managed disaster. All organizations involved in the community preparedness plan for mass casualties, including hospitals, need to agree in advance on who will serve as the single, regional spokesperson. See Appendix D for instructions to follow in light of an anthrax threat.

Use of a community-wide spokesperson will minimize disruption within hospitals if the press events are conducted away from healthcare facilities and use regularly scheduled and pre-announced media briefing times.

All organizations participating in the community preparedness plan will facilitate communications and reduce disruption of their own staffs if the plan for a pre-arranged community spokesperson also clearly identifies what others are *not* to say.

Hospitals often have established relationships with the local health reporters. In a mass casualty incident, the health reporter may not be the prime media contact. The government reporter, or crime reporter in the case of terrorism, may have the lead on the incident. The community spokesperson needs to be known and trusted by this reporter prior to any incident. Health experts who will be used to complement the spokesperson also should be known in advance to the reporter(s), if possible.

On alert: Who responds to bioterrorism?

If a bioterrorist attack should break out in your region, several different levels of bureaucracies get involved. The Model Emergency Response Communications Plan, a May 2000 report of the Association of State and Territorial Directors of Health Promotion and Public Health Education (ASTDHPPHE), included the following list of players you should be aware of in the event of an attack. It's important for your facility to know which agencies have which responsibilities.

Local agencies

- Frontline health providers—Report infectious disease case information to local health agency.

- First responders—Fire, police, and EMS personnel relay information to health officials or to the incident commander, especially in the case of announced terrorist-related infectious disease outbreaks.

- Hospitals and laboratories—Report and refer suspicious specimens to higher-level laboratories at the local and/or state level.

- Local department officials—Report and refer case information to state health agencies. For small-scale outbreaks, local health directors may serve as primary media spokespersons or delegate this function to a public information officer. Health directors may give final approval to release of emergency information.

- Local school officials—Function as a local resource to support the response effort. May be called upon to disseminate information to school populations. (In very serious situations, they may assist with consequence management by helping to arrange mass care, since schools are often used for this purpose.)

- Local media outlets—May be called upon to cooperate in public education efforts. For example, the media may maintain advance emergency information packets for release at the request of local officials. Media organizations will likely seek to verify field reports of the emergency's development with health officials.

- Elected officials—Function primarily as recipients of information. May participate in press conferences, as well as the unified command system in the case of large-scale emergencies.

- Public information system—Media spokespersons representing law enforcement, elected officials, and other entities outside the public health system may participate in the joint information center (JIC) in the case of large-scale emergencies.

State players

- State health department (SHD) officer/director—Oversees activities of core public health working group during an emergency response. Assures coordination of health agency activities with the JIC and unified command (UC) system and serves as liaison with the governor, as necessary. May also review/approve all or select public communications.

- SHD public information officer—Is responsible for all media contact and public relations activities, including rumor control, release of health education information to the public and to health professionals, release of emergency response information, and so on. Consults with other SHD staff as necessary to assure that all materials are current and accurate. May be designated as lead public health representative to the JIC.

- SHD laboratory director—Informs lower-level laboratories to watch for suspicious specimens. Provides protocols for the isolation of specific organisms and the safety of laboratory personnel. Provides instructions for the shipping/handling of infectious agents. Provides chain of evidence form (to be used in criminal investigations).

- SHD epidemiologist—Directs disease surveillance statewide. Designs and implements the statewide program to locate diagnosed and undiagnosed cases of illness and coordinates efforts to identify the causative agent in suspected outbreaks. Coordinates epidemiologic investigations with clinical laboratories and infection control practitioners statewide. Advises hospital infection control personnel and local health officials on information pertinent to public health, including protocols for disease investigation, control, and treatment. Notifies healthcare practitioners and, when appropriate, notifies or coordinates the notification of those affected by the disease. Communicates with and requests assistance as required from other SHD epidemiologists and the Centers for Disease Control (CDC). Updates the public information officer and other core working group members on the nature and scope of the outbreak and likely routes of transmission. Develops and implements public information programs for mass media distribution, including fact sheets for health education and public affairs staff within the health agency, and for Web site posting and press releases. Represents the health agency as required in public forums, including press and media briefings.

- SHD environmental health official—Serves as liaison with local environmental health staff and with the state and/or U.S. Department of Agriculture. May oversee collection of pathogen samples, especially when water- or food-borne.

- SHD emergency medical services agency—Supports regional EMS offices and local EMS agencies. Specific functions are similar to those of the SHD laboratory and SHD environmental health division.

- District/regional health officer—Serves as local public health contact. May designate local public affairs spokespersons in consultation with state staff. (Note: A variety of state public health organizational structures exist. For example, the state health department may also serve as a local health department. Therefore, a chain of communication from the state to the local level must be determined in advance.)

- Department of Agriculture—Is responsible for food inspections. Coordinates public education activities with health department staff and the JIC.

- State educational official—Functions as a state resource to support the response effort. May be called upon to disseminate information to school populations (especially if a university has inadvertently released a biological agent in the course of research activities). May also be called upon to help arrange mass care, since schools are often used for this purpose.

- Elected officials (political)—Function primarily as recipients of information. The governor signs the declaration of a regional or state emergency, designates someone from his or her office (usually a press secretary) to participate in the JIC, and, if necessary, requests that the president declare a national emergency. The governor may choose to participate in press conferences, as well as the UC system, in the case of large-scale emergencies.

- State press officers—Serve as liaisons to the JIC on behalf of the governor. (Note: All state and federal staff work to support local players.)

Federal players

- CDC—Upon request, CDC staff provide states with backup assistance in many areas, including data analysis, laboratory support, and public communications/education. If necessary, CDC will send communications staff and/or other experts on-site to provide assistance. Generally, CDC strives to coordinate its activities with states. The agency also conducts national surveillance activities and alerts states if worrisome trends become apparent. CDC facilitates the Health Alert Network (HAN) for information technology assessment, development, and enhancement. Either independently or in collaboration with states, CDC conducts extensive research activities and often issues national announcements with regard to research findings. CDC has quarantine power over ports of entry.

- U.S. Department of Agriculture—Involved in cases of agricultural bioterrorism or large-scale foodborne outbreaks. May provide laboratory backup and serve as a press liaison to the JIC.

- Food and Drug Administration—Involved in food- or water-borne outbreaks. May also be involved providing information on the availability of vaccines.

- National Institutes of Health—Supports laboratory diagnostics and conducts research to determine the sensitivity/resistance of the infectious agent to therapeutic antibiotics.

Terrorism: Keeping workers safe

Decontamination of patients is not just a matter of treating those patients, but also involves keeping your workers and hospital safe from contamination, which are requirements of both JCAHO and the Occupational Safety and Health Administration (OSHA).

Henry J. Siegelson, MD, FACEP, of Disaster Planning International and Emory University Department of Emergency Medicine in Atlanta, GA, said hospitals should keep in mind that numerous hazardous chemicals are stored, manufactured, transported, and utilized within the areas of most hospitals. Furthermore, hospitals should be ready in case of an accident at home or work, an industrial or transportation accident, or a terrorist attack.

Siegelson, who spoke at the June 2000 American Society of Healthcare Engineering conference in Seattle, WA, said facilities should, at the very least, be prepared to handle at least one patient exposed to a hazardous material. "If the hospital can function and deliver care to a single patient, then the policies can be easily configured to manage 10, 30, or even 100 patients," Siegelson said.

Decontaminating the patient

It is very difficult to determine exactly what a victim has been exposed to moments after an attack. Staff members will probably be running out to treat patients, not knowing the extent of their injuries or what the element was that caused those injuries. But before entering a hospital, the patients must be cleansed to prevent cross-contamination, Siegelson said.

"At the hospital, you have to be prepared for the unknown chemical," Siegelson said. "There are no shortcuts, because we're dealing with people's lives."

The level of decontamination depends on the type of exposure the victim suffers. If you are sure that a victim was exposed only to fume or vapor and is not symptomatic, then Siegelson said removing the patient's clothing is sufficient. If there is liquid or visible contamination or if the patient is symptomatic, then further steps must be taken, such as high-volume showering, possibly with soap.

After an explosive event, patients' clothing should be placed in a paper bag, transferred to a plastic bag, and then placed in a second plastic bag. After a chemical event, only plastic bags are required, Siegelson said. You should bag jewelry, keys, wallets, and purses separately from the clothes, and each should be tagged to identify the bag with the particular victim. Siegelson added that decontamination on hospital grounds is easier when done outside with sturdy, disposable, portable systems. If you use a permanent indoor system, it could get costly and require extensive engineering.

Protective equipment

When dealing with decontamination, it is important not only to ensure that the victim does not contaminate the facility, but also to protect the workers trying to treat the victim. Siegelson said that, in industrial situations with a known contaminant, a Level C suit may be sufficient.

However, with unknown chemicals or contaminants, your staff should be wearing a higher-level (Level B) suit.

Stanley "Skeet" Dickinson, an emergency medical technician and a hospital hazardous materials (HAZMAT) specialist in Carmel, IN, added that, before purchasing a protective suit, organizations should evaluate the product and its chemical degradation. For example, the seams should be made well and reveal no visible threads. You should be able to cover the zipper with a flap. The gloves, Dickinson added, should be one-size-fits-all, and the overboots should fit over most street shoes.

Siegelson suggested that radiation monitoring equipment be accessible at the emergency department (ED) triage area. Checking for radioactive contamination should be part of a routine procedure during such an event. You should take an "all-hazards approach" when choosing protective gear. Protect yourself against agents most commonly found in the community, Dickinson and Siegelson added.

Decontamination area

Dickinson offered the following advice on how to properly set up a decontamination area outside your facility:

1. **Secure the area.** Block and/or lock all entrances to the hospital except the ED entrance. Narrowing access reduces the risk of contaminating the facility.

2. **Set down a 16-foot by 20-foot tarp.** The tarp's purpose is more to denote the decontamination area than to provide chemical resistance. Keep staff members who are not wearing protective equipment away from the outlined area.

3. **Set up your portable shower system in one corner of the area.** Keep the shower raised so that the contaminated water is collected.

Water and electricity should obviously be piped into the area in that same corner as needed. Dickinson calls this the "warm and dirty" side.

4. **Have the incident commander supervise.** The person designated as the incident commander should observe the decontamination process from the "cold and clean" corner of the area.

5. **Undress patients.** Have people disrobe on the warm and dirty side and have blankets available for them as they wait to enter the shower. Provide as much privacy for the patients as possible. People might hesitate to disrobe if they cannot do so in private. Once they have disrobed, give them a blanket to keep warm until they can get into the shower.

6. **Dry the patients.** As patients emerge from the shower, have staff members ready with towels to dry them. Then give them new blankets to keep them warm. Have a container ready to collect the towels. Have HAZMAT team members ready to cover the patients with new blankets.

7. **Triage the patients.** Members of the ED should be waiting on the cold and clean side of the designated area, ready to take the decontaminated patients into the facility for treatment.

Chapter Two

Domestic Terrorism

Disaster plans meld distinct elements of security and credentialing

Hospitals dealing with the World Trade Center disaster saw volunteers and medical staff members come out in droves to offer assistance to emergency department (ED) trauma teams. The benefits of so much good will are obvious, but the back side of it is that sometimes too many people hurt—rather than help—disaster response coordination.

In the hours after the planes hit the towers, it was simply too crowded in Long Island College Hospital's (LICH) ED, says Lewis Kohl, MD, chairman of the department.

In addition to volunteers, even regular staff members were a burden, Kohl adds. Medical students came down to aid, and even though they meant well, they and others bogged down the emergency room.

"I had so many people in the emergency department that we couldn't move," Kohl says. "I literally stood in the emergency department and directed traffic. I spent a ridiculous amount of time moving people around."

Remember, if you have predetermined assignments for overflow help, such as through an incident command system, you may be able to better direct people to needed jobs. That way, if the urology team comes down to the emergency room to help during a disaster response—even though they probably won't be involved in the direct care of incoming casualties—they won't be just sitting around while trauma units work on patients.

Granted, this all depends on the size of your hospital's roster. A small community hospital may welcome help from any and all clinical staff.

Who comes in?

Adding to the confusion at LICH was that some security officers did not feel empowered to limit access to the emergency department, Kohl says. For example, an officer was unlikely to stop a doctor from entering, even if the physician might not have been needed inside.

St. Vincent's Manhattan Hospital instituted a lockdown of the property once the emergency plan activated. "We, in essence, had to concentrate on patrolling the ED," says safety officer Yvonne Wojcicki. "We pretty much shut down all the doors into the building except the main entrance and the ED entrance."

The hospital's security officers thoroughly checked staff identifications, and if someone didn't have a badge, [he or she] didn't get in, Wojcicki says.

Kohl wants to amend his facility's disaster plan by implementing a color code system that will help determine who gains entry into a busy ED during a disaster response. He envisions something as simple as a blue dot on identification badges for those employees who are allowed to go in, so security can easily keep track of the situation.

Sites deal with credentialing

There were many published stories about how doctors visiting New York and Washington stopped what they were doing and headed to the nearest hospital to offer their help after the attacks.

That creates a headache for credentialing these physicians—in other words, making sure they really are qualified to practice medicine. The dilemma is that during a disaster response, you don't want to spend a lot of time checking the backgrounds of people who are needed for patient care.

LICH used the Internet as part of its emergency credentialing procedure to check the credentials and state licensure of any doctor who volunteered.

North General Hospital in Manhattan was another hospital that readied itself for a wave of volunteer physicians. "Our [hospital has] a policy as part of our overall disaster plan that allows us to credential physicians who aren't on our medical staff by simply verifying their license and checking a positive photo ID," says Nilda Conrad, MBA, CMSC, CPCS, director of medical staff services.

North General also asks for a list of the physician's past hospital affiliations, but Conrad explains that sometimes there isn't time to call and verify each one. "We do the best we can, but if we're in a situation where hundreds of patients are flooding in, we have to let physicians help them," she says.

"After the World Trade Center collapsed, we received only 25 to 30 injured—we had expected to get many more," she adds. As a result, North General didn't need the assistance of any volunteer physicians and didn't enact its emergency credentialing policy after all.

Some hospitals require an administrator or high-level manager to sign off on emergency credentials; if that's the case in your facility, make sure that manager is in the disaster command center so he or she can easily be tracked down for signatures.

Phone coverage suffers

As soon as the attacks occurred, many phone providers in the New York area were swamped with people trying to contact family and friends. Some systems went down, including cell phone systems, Kohl says.

He believes nearly everyone in the city tried to use a phone at around the time of the attacks, which locked up communications for hospitals and other rescue services. LICH's emergency phone system worked, but cell phone coverage was nonexistent.

"If your disaster plan requires you to rely on cell phones as a backup, it's a bad plan," Kohl says. "I think we should purchase a couple of satellite phones just so we can be independent of our local [coverage] grid."

However, some hospitals have found cell phones to be very useful when entire building communications systems go down, such as during a flood of a hospital in Colorado last year.

Success and new challenges for hospitals at "ground zero"

Rush of volunteers and donations test plans

Shortly after the first plane crashed into the World Trade Center on September 11, hospitals in the New York City area implemented their disaster plans in anticipation of massive casualties.

Sadly, many victims never made it to the treatment rooms, but for the hospitals involved, there was some comfort in knowing their emergency management plans functioned well.

"[Our plan] worked better than we could have hoped," says Lewis Kohl, MD, chairman of the emergency department at Long Island College Hospital (LICH) in Brooklyn. LICH sits across the East River from Manhattan, and those who were there during the terrorist assault could see the World Trade Center towers burning across the water.

About 30 blocks from "ground zero," staff members at St. Vincent's Manhattan Hospital cleared their emergency department and prepared areas for overflow patients—a key point in their disaster plan.

Officials at the two hospitals say that, despite the success of the plans, they'll need to make some improvements. Here are three areas that they recommend safety committees look at while reassessing their emergency response policies:

Have an idea of what you want staff members to do during an emergency

The attacks occurred during a time when LICH was fully staffed, which meant many workers came to the emergency department looking for something to do. The hospital recently implemented a Hospital Emergency Incident Command System (HEICS). HEICS establishes a chain of command, assigns positions to a command post, and gives people in those positions job checklists to follow during a disaster.

Despite what many might think, staff members were not in a frenzy about the nearby terror. "No one panicked," Kohl says. "Everyone was basically looking for something to do." If they don't get a task to accomplish, people tend to get frustrated or angry, he adds, so have a list of jobs—even easy ones—that people can take up. Ideas include answering phones, transporting patients, or checking on incoming doctors' credentials.

St. Vincent's also uses an incident command system as part of its disaster plan, says safety officer Yvonne Wojcicki. Once the plan went into effect, the hospital's largest boardroom transformed into a command center, with the facility's president at the helm to assess department operations.

About 50 patients showed up at LICH's emergency department in the first hour after the attacks on the towers. A typical day sees 150 people come in to the emergency room. Initially, the hospital revved up to handle

50 patients per hour for two days, but that turned out not to be necessary, Kohl says.

"When the Trade Center collapsed, the casualties just stopped," he says.

Wojcicki echoes those thoughts, saying that, as of September 28, a total of only 673 patients from the attacks came in; 112 of them were admitted. Saint Clare's Health Services in Denville, NJ, implemented its disaster plan at its four campuses because of its proximity to New York and in response to orders from the governor of New Jersey, says Robert Westenberger, MCO, corporate director of safety and regulatory compliance.

"We had been told that we would see upwards of 200 to 300 people, although in the end we saw four walk-ins. We did set up a decontamination [area] due to the asbestos exposure on clothes [from the towers collapsing]," adds Westenberger, who served as the incident commander once the facility began disaster operations.

Have a procedure to handle volunteers

Following the attacks, New York residents took volunteering to new heights, which had some repercussions.

"Usually you don't think you're going to have enough help or you'll be overwhelmed," Kohl says. The fact is, LICH truly was inundated—by people who showed up offering assistance.

"We needed more people to handle the volunteers" than the clinical duties, he says. Your disaster plans should state who will deal with overflow volunteers and where you'll direct them.

"We could never have planned on the volunteers and turnout we got, and that's something we're going to have to look at as we go forward," Wojcicki says.

In fact, too many people were ready for duty who didn't have much to do. "We were literally outside our emergency department waiting," she adds. LICH asked many volunteers who simply weren't needed to instead give blood at the New York City Blood Bank, but even that site had too many people by the first day.

Know what you'll do with donations

St. Vincent's didn't fully anticipate how much equipment and goods people would provide to the hospital, Wojcicki says.

"We had donated clothes that were piling up on us," she says. "We had to step back and say, 'How are we going to control this?' "

St. Vincent's logged in donated goods and distributed them to all treatment areas within the hospital, as well as to rescue crews at the towers.

"Most of the used clothing from community residents was placed in our clothing room," Wojcicki says. "The packaged items, such as sweat socks and T-shirts, were sent to the [disaster] scene." Staff members sent other donations to organizations such as the American Red Cross and the Salvation Army.

At one point on September 11, as St. Vincent's clinical staff members waited outside the emergency department for victims, a truck pulled up unannounced and dropped off 24 wheelchairs for the hospital to use.

The donation was great, but it also alarmed Wojcicki and others; the fact that the truck pulled up so close to the building raised worries about security and access to the hospital. No one knew whether more terrorism was on the way.

Chapter Three

Fires

Plane crash: Expect the unexpected

Hospital staff often train for responding to emergencies (a car crash, a train wreck, even the possibility of an infectious outbreak) outside of their facility. But what about when an emergency occurs *at* your facility? When a plane crashed through the roof of Midwestern Regional Medical Center in Zion, IL, on February 8, 2000, staff members were ready.

What happened?

Midwestern Regional is about two miles from an airport. On February 8, two small planes collided in the air, sending one crashing through the roof and into the top-floor boardroom of the hospital's five-story tower.

The fifth floor of the tower does not have patient rooms, but it does have physical therapy rooms, a cardiopulmonary unit, offices, the executive boardroom, and the engineering department. The second through fourth floors house patient care areas, including the bone marrow transplant unit.

Three people died in the crash: the pilot and passenger of the plane that hit the roof, and the pilot of the other plane, which crashed into a nearby neighborhood. Also, 13 hospital employees suffered injuries, the most severe being burns. None of the 32 patients in the hospital was injured.

Immediate response

Soon after the plane crashed through the roof and into the boardroom on the fifth floor (snapping an 18-inch I-beam in the building's framework) fuel from the aircraft began leaking and then exploded, causing a fire. The building's sprinkler system came on, while the air-handling system shut down as designed.

Within a minute, administrators made the decision to evacuate the entire building, says Anne Meisner, vice president of patient care services at the hospital. Staff members helped patients down the stairs from the upper floors to a triage unit set up in the emergency room (ER).

Following a community-based emergency plan shared by Midwestern Regional and surrounding hospitals, staff members evacuated patients from the building according to immediate needs. Patients from the bone marrow transplant unit were the first to exit the building; neighboring healthcare sites provided the special housing areas these patients needed to survive. Additionally, an area of the ER was designated for the bone marrow patients.

Meanwhile, respiratory employees shut off the medical gas units on the fifth floor. Upon arrival, fire authorities recommended shutting off the gases to the third and fourth floors as a precaution, but allowed gas systems on the first and second floors to remain on, says Jerry Butts, director of cardiopulmonary services.

One oversight in the hospital's emergency plan was that the ER did not have enough portable oxygen tanks available in case the entire building's medical gas system needed to be shut down. In response, staff members had to bring a tank from the fifth floor down to the ER.

Fire contained, but damage results

Sprinklers and firefighters helped contain the blaze to the impact area, Kramer says. "There was no fire damage in any other part of the hospital," she explains. "The fire was contained to the impact area . . . The hospital did suffer damage, mostly from water, from our own sprinkler system."

Manpower was not a problem, because the accident happened during a shift change, so about 300 of the hospital's 455 employees were in the hospital when the plane crashed, Meisner says.

The hospital does not use the Incident Command System (ICS) as described in National Fire Protection Association (NFPA) 99, Healthcare Facilities. However, the facility does use a similar hierarchy that establishes a chain of command.

When fire authorities arrived, they and hospital administrators set up a joint command post, where they were able to make joint decisions and coordinate tasks, Meisner notes. Also, requests from the media for information came in droves once word got out about the crash.

Prior drills prepare staff

Even in the chaos, patient evacuation went quickly and staff members remained calm, Kramer says. She attributes the ease of the evacuation to prior fire and emergency drills.

"We drill every department . . . every quarter, for every shift," she says. That fire drill schedule follows standards from the Joint Commission. JCAHO requires emergency drills to be held semi-annually.

"They are unannounced drills," Kramer adds. In the administration's eyes, the drills count as important ongoing training, and with the plane crash, the rewards of drilling were self-evident.

"There is a lot of value in practicing and imagining scenarios, and working them through," adds Meisner, who thinks drill performance will improve even more because of the crash.

Additionally, all new employees at the facility receive two days, worth of safety training during orientation, as well as department-specific training. Each employee also takes part in a mandatory refresher course each year.

Training strategies

The facility posts evacuation routes throughout the hospital, but the *Life Safety Code®* doesn't require such postings (although any facility is free to go beyond code minimums). The routes are posted in common rooms and by elevators, and Midwestern Regional trains its employees to recognize the routes, says Debbie Horton, safety coordinator for the hospital.

Staff members also get trained on the Rescue, Alarm, Confine, Extinguish (RACE) strategy. During fire drills, coordinators use real people as mock patients so that employees learn what it's like to have to physically move people to different smoke compartments or even down stairs, Horton adds. That part of the training became particularly important after the plane crash, because six patients were nonambulatory and had to be carried on blankets to lower floors.

Access to the building

The hospital's general policy is to have employees wear identification tags (IDs) at all times, but having IDs became extremely important after the crash. The fire department and Midwestern Regional's security officers strictly controlled access to the hospital, so that only employees who had valid ID badges could get back into the building.

Susan Thomas, the hospital's director of human resources, says building access falls under fire and emergency drill procedures. During a fire or disaster, two to four employees must guard all entrances. The idea is not only to stop unwanted visitors from entering, but also to protect employees who might otherwise enter an unsafe building.

Furthermore, Midwestern Regional needed to ensure that people did not go into the building and perhaps get injured by an unstable part of the structure or damaged equipment.

"We weren't sure . . . how much damage had occurred and what potential there was for subsequent damage," Kramer explains.

Aftermath of the crash

A large concern after the crash was hazardous contamination due to the gas leak and fire. The hospital hired a disaster recovery company to check out the air handlers for contamination. The company cleaned the handlers, tested the equipment, and also monitored the air quality in the hospital.

No major plan changes

There is no plan to rewrite the facility's disaster plan to specifically mention plane crashes, and training will probably remain the same.

"As for the safety orientation, I don't think we'll change anything, other than we'll now say we've been through this, we know this works, and these are the reasons why," Thomas says.

In the days following the crash, a child in the lobby of one of the hospital's buildings accidentally pulled a fire alarm station. Staff members quickly went into action, unsure of whether their facility was facing another emergency. The employees' immediate response conveyed the awareness they had learned as a result of the plane crash.

"We learned to take all drills seriously," Butts says. "Everyone in the department knows you never know when a disaster will strike. We have a new sense of urgency."

Fatal fire in Virginia

On December 31, 1994, a fire broke out in a patient's room at Southside Regional Medical Center in Petersburg, VA. Five patients died. Smoke and flames severely damaged an area of the hospital, and staff members faced the difficult task of finding out what went wrong at the 468-bed site.

What happened?

On the day of the fire, a patient became increasingly agitated and was eventually restrained by the hands and feet. At 9:06 p.m., a nurse heard a noise, looked into the patient's room, and saw the bed and cubicle curtain in flames.

The nurse closed the door, went into the hall, and pulled the alarm station. She called for more help and went back to the room with a blanket. She tried to smother the flames and got one leg restraint free before the intensity of the smoke drove her and other nurses out of the room.

Smoke spread through the ceiling and acoustic tile into adjoining rooms. In the room of origin, the heat melted an oxygen wall unit, allowing the gas to flow into the room. At one point, the fire shattered an outside window to the room, feeding an air supply to the flames.

Closing the door

Patricia Spacek, RN, MPS, and director of risk management, said her staff never determined whether the nurse fully closed the door to the room of origin when the fire drove them out. "Whether or not it was closed completely and came back open when the fire blew out the window, we don't know," Spacek said.

However, the (NFPA concluded that the nurse did not close the door. The patient in the room of origin died of injuries from the fire. Four other patients died of smoke inhalation. Investigators determined that smoke spread through the suspended ceilings because the walls between the patient sleeping rooms did not extend up to the ceiling slab. The *Life Safety Code* (*LSC*) doesn't require separation protection between patient rooms.

Notification problems

The central alarm company did not respond to the initial pull station alarm when it came in at 9:06 p.m. because the alarm system was partly disabled due to an ongoing renovation project. This delayed the notification to the fire department until the hospital's switchboard operator called 911 five minutes later.

Other factors that aided the fire's spread were that smoke detectors were not in the patient rooms and sprinklers did not protect the area. The *LSC* does not automatically require sprinklers in existing healthcare facilities, nor does it require smoke detectors in patient rooms. Since then, Southside has spent $1.8 million to install a full sprinkler system and has also reworked its alarms to avoid future notification problems.

Busy hours

Spacek said every facility needs to plan for emergency response when the hospital is busy. The day of Southside's fire was New Year's Eve on a Saturday night, which meant staff members were very busy attending to patients and visitors in the emergency room.

The preparedness plan should include provisions for emergencies that occur on nights, weekends, or holidays. The plan also needs to detail who is in charge if there is an emergency and how quickly top management can get to the hospital during a crisis.

"I ask you to go back to your facility and ask yourself, 'Does [my plan] really work?' " Spacek said.

And the policy says . . .

Spacek provided a backbone approach to analyzing a preparedness plan. A facility's policies and procedures should include the following:

- What you intended to write
- What you actually wrote
- What you intended to teach
- What you actually taught
- What the staff actually does
- What outside parties will read from the policies

The last item is particularly important because lawyers, reporters, and surveyors are not always familiar with hospital procedures or lingo.

"I suggest [that you] look at your policies very critically. Ask a friend to look at them and see if they make sense," Spacek explained.

Spacek also said managers should check their state laws to learn what a facility must turn over to surveyors, police, and attorneys, and determine whether this information has to be in writing or can be given verbally. Also check on who has authority to take photographs.

Restraint policy

After the fire, administrators reviewed the facility's restraint policy, and, since the incident, restraint use has declined at the hospital. Spacek said staff members now try to be more "restraint appropriate" when dealing with difficult patients, and there is also more interaction with personnel from the medical-psychiatric unit.

The local fire department was unable to determine the cause of the fire. However, investigators speculated that the fire started when the patient in the room tried to smoke in bed while restrained.

Fire crews found the charred remnants of matches and cigarettes on the floor of the room. Investigators never resolved how the patient (a former nurse undergoing treatment) got the smoking materials while in restraints, the *Richmond Times Dispatch* reported in March 1998.

According to Spacek, 12 lawsuits related to the fire were resolved out of court.

Roof fire in Missouri

Even something as mundane as getting a building's roof repaired can have serious potential consequences from a life safety standpoint. Take the case of Children's Mercy Hospital, a 177-bed facility in Kansas City, MO, that was 90% occupied with patients on January 28, 1999, when a fire broke out on the rooftop.

There were no injuries during the fire, although staff members evacuated patients from the five-story hospital to the outside. The top floor sustained water and smoke damage.

Roof tar suspected

Local authorities believe new tarring on the roof, which had just been laid by a contractor that day, somehow accidentally ignited.

"The fire never entered the building at any time. It [remained] on the roof," says Jonathan Lowe, community relations assistant at the hospital.

Roofing work with tar usually involves propane-heated kettles that warm the tar. Tar work and welding are common causes of building fires, due to the heat involved.

Lowe says the contractor did observe a 30-minute fire watch after the day's work was over, but during that time no one on the work crew detected anything unusual on the roof or saw anything smoldering. The fire was reported about four hours after the work crew left.

Evacuation planning

Staff members at Children's Mercy participate in emergency preparedness drills twice a year, including evacuation scenarios, and officials credit these practice runs for employee readiness when the real thing occurred.

"We find [drills] are very important," says Lowe. The staff's response to the fire "went as smoothly as it did because we do practice."

Employees performed an evacuation of 60 patients from their rooms to the outside during the fire, Lowe adds. Staff members brought many of the patients back inside after a short time. (See Appendix F for questions regarding fire drills.)

Defend in place

Most healthcare facilities endorse defend-in-place strategies in the event of a fire, where complete evacuation is kept to a minimum, and patients and staff in the immediate area of a fire instead move to a safe, adjacent smoke compartment within the hospital.

The *LSC* requires that a facility's evacuation procedures be part of its emergency preparedness plan; however, there are no requirements in either the *LSC* or NFPA 99, Standard for Healthcare Facilities, that mandate specific types of evacuations.

In commentary for both the *LSC* and the *Healthcare Facilities Handbook,* the NFPA suggests that defend-in-place strategies are the ideal response when a fire breaks out, but not the only option.

"It should again be noted that while movement (particularly evacuation to the outside) is the least desired action for a healthcare facility to take, it may be necessary in some disasters," the *Healthcare Facilities Handbook* states in appendix note C-11.3.3. "A facility needs to be prepared for situations when total evacuation is necessary," such as fire, a tornado, or any other man-made or natural disaster.

In the plan

Lowe says the emergency disaster plan at Children's Mercy requires staff members to evacuate patients outdoors. According to Lowe, he and others at Children's Mercy have heard about defend-in-place strategies that other facilities use, and he expects his hospital will review the provisions of its emergency plan concerning outdoor evacuation during an alarm.

"I think that [policy] is something we may reevaluate," he says, adding that a fluid emergency plan that can adapt to a given fire situation might work better than a rigid plan that mandates all evacuations must go to the outside of the building.

Lowe thinks that in this case, however, going outdoors was prudent, because alarms went off and no one initially knew the location of the fire or source of the alarms. "[Staff members] were trying to find out exactly where the fire was," he explains.

Other fire safety experts say that, in some cases, it may be more dangerous to take patients outside a building, particularly if the fire is outside.

Quick-hit reviews

Apart from drills, employees wear constant reminders of fire alarm response procedures. In addition to the identification badges that they must wear at all times, personnel also carry a card that lists Children's Mercy's mission statement and procedures to follow if there is a fire.

Among the steps listed on the card is a review of:

- Fire protection acronyms such as SAFE (Sound the Alarm, Fight the fire, Evacuate the patients) and PASS (portable fire extinguisher training that stands for Pull, Aim, Squeeze, Sweep)
- Emergency telephone numbers for the safety, security, and engineering offices
- The code word for a fire in the building (for example, "Doctor Red") and how to use it

Damage and the aftermath

When you look at fire drills and disaster planning, make sure to consider the aftermath, particularly whether your facility is prepared to handle cleanup of smoke stains, odors, pools of water, and drenched carpeting.

Cleanup went smoothly at Children's Mercy, thanks to a dedicated team that quickly went into action. A 22-member night crew, including personnel from the environmental services department, worked overnight to clean up the damaged areas. Within 24 hours of the fire, the facility reopened all but the most damaged areas. The hospital never fully closed down in the fire's aftermath.

Environmental services employees cleaned room walls, carpets, drapes, and cubicles, and also used a special chemical to remove smoke odors, Lowe says. The crews "really came through," he adds.

Lowe estimates the fire caused from $200,000 to $500,000 worth of damage. "Most of the damage sustained in the hospital was water damage from the fire crews," he explains.

In Dallas, fire drills pay off

A roof fire that occurred on July 26, 2000, at Children's Medical Center of Dallas, TX, offered some valuable lessons in fire drill preparation and construction project safeguards. The fire necessitated horizontal evacuations on three patient care floors, but there were no patient injuries, and employees responded well when a "code red" page went out, says Greg Terrell, MS, CSP, ARM, director of risk management and safety officer at the 322-bed pediatric hospital.

"All of our fire drills really paid off," Terrell says. "People knew what to do with the evacuation. Everyone was rocking and rolling." (See Appendix G for tips on evacuation drills.)

What happened?

Children's Medical Center was in the midst of a construction project that was adding several stories to part of the building to match the height of an existing tower. When the project was done, the addition would connect to the tower. As part of the work, contractors were removing the tower's pre-cast concrete "skin," which exposed the building.

Crews used a propane torch for some of their work. At the end of the day, the workers shut off their equipment and went home. Unbeknownst to them, the torch work ignited some wood on the roof, and a fire broke out after the contractors left.

A hospital engineering employee was repairing a rooftop air conditioning unit at a building across the street when he saw flames on the top of the nearby facility. The employee called central dispatch to report the fire, which in turn informed the security department. Security members subsequently pulled the fire alarm and had a "code red" page announced at 5:17 p.m., which informed employees of a potential fire and the location.

Terrell says that Children's Medical Center has a fire response team (made up of the administrator on call, engineering, a nursing administrative supervisor, security, and respiratory care) that immediately responds to a code red to see whether there really is a fire or whether it is a less serious incident, such as someone burning popcorn or a child pulling the alarm. If the alarm is legitimate, the code is paged again.

The fire response team made its way to the roof to combat the fire. At the same time, smoke had crept into the building through cracks in the building's exterior, which had been exposed by the contractor work. The smoke, which evaded temporary sealed dust partitions put up by the contractors to keep construction dust away from patient care areas, went above ceiling tiles and into open plenums.

Evacuation

The three floors immediately below the roof contain care areas for hematology, oncology, orthopedic services, asthma, and bone marrow transplants, and many of these areas house immuno-compromised children, Terrell explains. Because of the sensitive nature of their health, once the smoke came in, a decision was quickly made to evacuate patients on those three floors horizontally to safe waiting areas in an adjacent tower.

"It was definitely the smoke that was causing us to evacuate," Terrell says. The response of the employees was rapid. Within 10 minutes, staff members relocated 49 patients. "I was extremely pleased about that," he says.

Meanwhile, the fire response team members quickly extinguished the fire on the roof. The fire department arrived soon after and tended to hot spots to make sure they were out. About 45 minutes later, patients from the fifth floor were allowed to return to their rooms, since they were orthopedic patients who weren't as sensitive to the smoke's remnants. By 7 p.m., patients from the fourth floor (asthma patients) returned to their rooms, and patients from the sixth floor (hematology and oncology patients) came back by 9 p.m. Employees used particulate air monitoring to make sure it was safe to return to the evacuated areas.

RCAF

Terrell says the hospital's employees came through during a difficult time when lives were at risk, and he credits fire drill training as the prime reason for that success. During drills, employees are quizzed on a procedure called "RCAF," which is similar to the RACE strategy. Terrell says RCAF stands for the following:

R—Rescue the patients
C—Confine the fire
A—Alert others about the fire
F—Fight the fire

Terrell urges other facilities to keep up with required drills, because it helps with employee preparation. "Sometimes you think people aren't paying attention to code red drills, but they are," he says.

What could have been better?

One area Terrell feels could be improved upon is the decision to implement an internal disaster plan when a situation warrants an evacuation. He believes that once the evacuation was deemed necessary, the facility should have paged an internal disaster code, which would have set up a command center, activated an employee pool from which to draw extra help, and established a media relations post.

"When it gets to the point where [you need] an evacuation, it needs to be done via an internal disaster plan," Terrell says. "In this situation, there was no harm, no foul, because everyone was fine." But if the fire had been more serious, a command center would have made it easier to manage the incident.

Marking patient room doors

Staff members were not trained to mark off closed patient room doors during an evacuation to let others know that the rooms were empty, which is an aspect of training that will change, Terrell says. During the evacuation, employees ended up double-checking some of the rooms because it was not clear whether the rooms were empty. Again, that situation was not a problem this time, but it is easy to think of other scenarios where staff members would be racing to clear an area, Terrell adds.

Terrell says the facility will establish a policy on how to properly mark empty patient care rooms. Some suggestions that Children's Medical Center is considering include putting a pillow at the base of the closed door or sticking a temporary decal on the door once a staff member has checked the room.

Increased walk-throughs

The fire caused Children's Medical Center and the construction contractor to rethink strategies for keeping a closer eye out for the problems that can occur when hot work, such as the use of propane torches, is done. The contractor had the proper permits for the work and the propane torch was shut off correctly, yet no one walked the construction site after the work crews left for the day to ensure everything was okay, Terrell says.

Since the fire, there has been "heightened awareness and cooperation with the contractors and Children's to make us aware of when and where they're doing hot work," Terrell says. Now, when work crews leave at the end of their shift, they inform the facility, and a member of the hospital's security team will inspect the site. In the past, security officers would walk the site at least twice every shift. "Now we know if there's hot work going on, we want to walk through every 15 to 30 minutes," Terrell says.

Access problems

Another problem did not become apparent until the fire department arrived: access to the building. The week the fire occurred, the main front entrance was closed due to the ongoing construction work. An alternative entrance was nearby, but firefighters did not know this until they arrived to respond to the roof blaze.

"To tell you the truth, the closure was thoroughly planned out. However, we didn't consider informing external agencies," Terrell acknowledges.

Some life safety experts believe that the situation may have been averted if Interim Life Safety Measures were implemented for the entrance. The access problem was a minor setback, as the other entrance was close by and the situation did not really hamper the fire department's efforts. But at the same, it would have made sense to let the fire department know of the change, Terrell says. "As a result of that, we have established enhanced communications with the fire department," he adds.

Soon after the fire, Children's Medical Center sent a letter of thanks to the fire chief for his crew's efforts and also invited senior fire officials to tour the hospital at some point to become more familiar with the building's setup. Terrell thinks this type of visit during normal operations will be of benefit in the event of another fire.

Chapter Four

Floods

As Houston facilities recover, they tell of flood lessons

Imagine that a nasty storm stalls over your city or town. Your healthcare facility loses main power, and backup generators begin working. You have 570 patients on 26 floors. But then, over the next six hours, the building progressively loses emergency power as two subbasements that contain much of your mechanical equipment flood.

Welcome to the world of St. Luke's Episcopal Hospital, one of the facilities in Houston devastated by floodwaters at the Texas Medical Center campus—ground zero for much of the damage from Tropical Storm Allison on June 8–10, 2001.

"By 7 o'clock in the morning [on June 9], we had lost everything. We were literally dead in the water," says Mike Reno, St. Luke's administrative director of support services. Through a dedicated, concerted effort among the community, vendors, and employees, the hospital reopened by June 20.

Judging from the Texas Medical Center's problems, other sites should complete a hazard vulnerability analysis that examines what high waters could do to their facilities, says Russell Phillips, president of Russell Phillips & Associates/MedSafe in Rochester, NY. Phillips visited some of the facilities in Houston shortly after the flooding in an educational research effort under the auspices of the NFPA.

Based on what they saw, Reno and Phillips suggest three broad areas to look at when planning disaster recovery policies:

1. Patient safety
2. Emergency plan details
3. Location of critical equipment

Patient safety

St. Luke's first subbasement contained anywhere from 4 in to 3.5 ft of water. In the second, lower subbasement, there was five to seven feet of flooding. Facilities in the Texas Medical Center were not designed to withstand that much water, Reno says.

Sensing the danger of total power loss, St. Luke's moved 54 critical patients through an enclosed walkway to an adjacent medical tower about 45 minutes before emergency power went out. In the tower, staff members turned an outpatient surgery center into a makeshift intensive care unit.

Workers also transferred some patients to nearby hospitals that still accepted incoming cases, though many patients stayed at St. Luke's while the utilities were off. Some power supplies, as well as heating and ventilation systems, were back on line within two days, Reno says.

"Our concern was . . . we had patients on ventilators and other mechanical equipment that needed power," he adds. "We maintained full emergency power at our medical tower," which only had 2 in of water on the lobby floor.

The successful transfers of patients was due in part to key people on site—such as the chief of staff and the chief quality officer—who were able to get accurate information and then make quick decisions. When facility workers told them emergency power was in jeopardy, the executives immediately ordered the transfer of particularly ill patients and obtained battery backup for others.

"I felt it was hectic, but never chaotic," Reno says. "Everyone kept their heads because we were able to stay focused on what was [most] important: protecting the patients—not making sure the building was okay."

There were no patient deaths attributable to the flood, Reno says. Patients died during that period, but the hospital says their medical conditions, not the disaster, led to their deaths.

Six patients died at The Methodist Hospital, which is also at the Texas Medical Center. The hospital says those patients were critical already and the flood did not contribute to their deaths, though at least one family publicly disputed that in the Houston Chronicle, arguing that the power loss increased the suffering of a relative who died.

(Meanwhile, the Texas Department of Human Services investigated the deaths of two assisted living residents involved in an evacuation.)

Emergency plan details

St. Luke's activated its emergency plan several days before the flooding because heavy rains had hit outlying areas, so the hospital needed to warn employees who lived in those areas about the problems. At that time, officials set up a 24-hour command center, and they kept the plan activated as the weather got worse near the facility. In the interim, the hospital opened dedicated communication lines, monitored satellite weather information, and contacted vendors, Reno says.

The emergency plan details staff responsibilities. During the policy's development, St. Luke's sought the opinions of all staff members, from physicians to housekeeping personnel.

"This is what set the foundation for us," Reno says. "[The emergency plan] wasn't perfect, and it can and will be improved . . . But because of the depth and breadth of people contributing to it, it was a tremendous resource."

While the facility never conducted an emergency drill for a flood scenario, it has done them for hurricanes, which helped employees better understand how to transfer and move patients, he adds. Also, a new medical building under construction by St. Luke's had a steam leak in March that required water removal and restoration, which turned out to be a good primer for what was to come during the flood.

However, there were noted problems with the emergency plan:

1. Officials relied too much on Internet access to weather updates, Reno says. When power failed, St. Luke's could not get the latest information or tell staff members the safest ways to get to or from work. The facility plans to install hard-wire landlines to the National Weather Service and the local emergency management office so it can maintain direct communication in the event of a future disaster.

2. The plan took for granted that executives responsible for implementing parts of the response would be able to get to St. Luke's, which was a bad assumption, Reno says. As a result, key players who were there juggled more duties than anticipated.

Listed below are additional problems that Houston medical facilities encountered during the floods. Emergency management plans should anticipate scenarios and recovery efforts dealing with the following conditions:

- Inability of staff members to communicate with each other in the hospital, and with outside people
- Failure of utilities such as power, gas, water, and sewer systems
- Lack of sufficient food and liquids for patients and employees
- Problems with doctors, nurses, and other personnel being able to get to the facility
- Malfunction of the heating, ventilation, and air conditioning units
- Troubles with pharmacy and laboratory services
- Physical damage to the structures of buildings

Source: Russell Phillips of Russell Phillips & Associates/MedSafe

Accreditation concerns

Emergency management plans, which the Joint Commission on Accreditation of Healthcare Organizations (JCAHO) requires, should address flood scenarios if a facility is in a flood-prone area.

The JCAHO also wants a healthcare facility to determine its role as part of any community disaster response plan, says John Murray, Jr., CHMM, CSP, safety director at Baystate Health System in Springfield, MA.

Looking at Houston's experience, it is easy to see how the lack of integration with the community—for example, in terms of the number of beds and intensive care units available at nearby hospitals—was a significant obstacle to the overall response, Phillips says. "They had to put it together during the disaster" with outside help from the Department of Veterans Affairs, he adds.

Location of critical equipment

Facilities should contact their local municipal or county engineer for help in determining the high water point in the facility, Phillips says.

If you determine that you have a flood threat, some mitigation solutions include putting the generator up on blocks or stilts tall enough to stay out of high waters, or relocating generator equipment to another floor. This is feasible in new construction but expensive in existing buildings because you may need to reinforce floors or lose patient care space, either of which could cost millions, Phillips says.

However, relocation comes with a price, Reno says. St. Luke's did not have its equipment above ground because it was cost-prohibitive to reinforce the structure to withstand the sheer weight of machinery and units.

"In 20-20 hindsight, it was not the best choice," says Reno. St. Luke's estimated total damage from the flood is $90.5 million.

Reno warns that once you move mechanical equipment above the 10th floor, you will probably double your reinforcement costs for every additional story. Also, what you may gain in flood protection by moving up, you could lose in terms of other risks, he adds. For example, winds can threaten generators on a roof.

However, heeding lessons learned during the flood, St. Luke's will rethink some equipment locations in its new building under construction. Officials had already planned to put vital equipment on the third floor, but now they will also likely install the generator pumps on that level to avoid floodwaters, Reno says.

Equipment at other facilities

Shriners Hospital for Children, also part of the Texas Medical Center, has no basement. Its critical equipment is above grade, which helped the facility, as did its location at the far southwest corner of the campus, where waters weren't quite as high, says Delbert Reed, SAM, CHUM, safety officer and director of clinical engineering and maintenance.

"If your gear is above grade one or two floors, you can still keep your critical systems going," Reed says. Shriners had only about $1,000 worth of damage, mostly from leaking ceiling tiles.

The Methodist Hospital lost its fire pumps and one building's switchgear equipment because the items were below grade. Emergency generators on the ground floor survived the flooding, says John Parker, CFEI, CHSP, fire safety representative.

Officials at Methodist plan to bring switchgear and communications equipment out of the lower levels. "A lot of offices will be relocated [to the basements]," Parker says. "We'll move conference rooms down to the basements."

The fire pumps will stay below ground, though, because of the difficulty in moving them. To compensate, the hospital plans to upgrade its flood protection downstairs. It already had flood logs and flood doors in place, but they couldn't withstand the rains from Tropical Storm Allison, Parker says.

Methodist, which suffered $300 million in losses, was scheduled to finally reopen its emergency room in mid-July 2001.

Houston waters cripple basement electrical systems

Perhaps the biggest early lesson coming out of the floods in Houston is that putting critical electrical equipment and emergency generators below grade poses a tremendous risk. Hospitals that took the biggest hits in the city were probably those whose electrical systems couldn't survive the rising waters.

Even before severe flooding overtook most of the Texas Medical Center, officials at the various hospitals in the campus were conducting a long-term hazard vulnerability analysis of potential water worries.

"We were asking hypothetically what would happen if there was a flood," says Delbert Reed, SAM, CHUM, safety officer and director of clinical engineering and maintenance at Shriners Hospital for Children, one the center's facilities.

Now, while recovering from the record-breaking washout June 8–10, the medical center is beginning to dissect what its hospitals learned as a way to prevent future catastrophes.

All power goes out

Hermann Memorial Hospital had to evacuate all 540 patients after normal and emergency power failed, according to the *Houston Chronicle.* Sensing the dangers early on, officials there decided to move about 50 critical patients through an enclosed walkway from Hermann to an adjacent medical tower just 30 minutes before backup power went out. Meanwhile, the hospital also suffered tremendous equipment damage, including on a floor where floodwaters destroyed cardiac diagnostic equipment valued at $60 million.

Some of Hermann's electrical system is below grade, and the floodwaters extensively damaged it, according to the hospital. Along with immediate repairs that were expected to keep the hospital closed until mid-July, Hermann indicates it will look at long-term plans to relocate electrical equipment to more appropriate spots.

"I think the people in the Texas Medical Center will revisit the location of their critical systems and distribution systems," Reed says. He thinks hospitals will look closely at isolating critical equipment in areas out of the basements.

"If your gear is above grade one or two floors, you can still keep your critical systems going," he says.

All medical centers should check their high water marks in the basements to make sure equipment won't be in danger, particularly emergency generators, says Russell Phillips, president of Russell Phillips & Associates/MedSafe in Rochester, NY. Phillips visited some of the devastated facilities in Houston shortly after the flooding.

Raise the equipment

Some solutions could include putting the generator up on blocks or stilts tall enough to stay out of high waters, or totally relocating generator equipment to another floor, Phillips says.

Facilities should contact their local municipal or county engineer for help in determining the high water mark in the basement, he adds.

Phillips also suggests conducting a hazard vulnerability analysis for the location of your generator. The analysis should "consider the high water mark, as is evidenced by the recent floods in Houston," he says.

Emergency management plans, which the Joint Commission on Accreditation of Healthcare Organizations requires, should address flood scenarios if a facility is in a flood-prone area. Last December 2000, a Colorado hospital lost its telecommunications systems for days after a flood destroyed phone equipment in the basement.

Communication bolsters efforts

Shriners suffered only about $1,000 in damage, mostly from two dozen water-soaked ceiling tiles. Compare that to the estimated $2 billion in losses that the entire medical center campus is facing, and you can see why Reed considers himself lucky.

Nonetheless, Reed says he was caught off-guard by some of the challenges of Tropical Storm Allison. For example, even though he lives only 12 miles from the facility, he could not get to the building at the height of the problems because of flooding in the Texas Medical Center.

His security staff members, who couldn't leave the building for the same reason, became his connection to what was going on. Communication skills were very important, as everyone had to listen well to each other and also provide reliable information, Reed says.

"Our staff did an outstanding job," he says. "The hospital as a whole pulled together to make sure patient safety wasn't compromised and the facility was maintained."

Dallas hospital copes with drenching disaster

It was like a scene out of a movie: Torrential rains flood the streets and parking lot around Baylor University Medical Center in Dallas, submerging cars and making travel impossible. Suddenly, the high water bursts through the automatic doors of the emergency department, flooding the area in two feet of water.

Hospital staff members scramble to move 35 patients and save what valuable equipment they can. Patients and family members panic, but staff members are able to relocate them all to the floor above only moments before the elevators shut down.

"Fortunately, being in the emergency department, the staff was able to think quickly," said Marguerite McCarthy, administrative director of the emergency department at Baylor. "They just worked very well together."

The flood hit Dallas on May 5, 1995, leaving many people homeless and killing 15 people in the city. Although it happened several years ago, the lessons learned from the disaster will stick with Baylor staff for years to come. In truth, the hospital wasn't prepared for a flash flood at its facility (after all, it seemed like an unlikely event), yet staff members performed admirably, McCarthy said.

A sea of troubles

When the water came crashing through the doors, the shift supervisor immediately alerted Baylor staff and the local police, McCarthy said. Staff rushed to get emergency department patients to higher ground (the post-anesthesia care unit directly above the department). It was about 10 p.m., so staff knew the unit would be empty. The move was a challenge for the medical center, where staff members are used to moving patients horizontally—that is, relocating them to somewhere else on the same floor or level. But because water was rushing in, patients were moved vertically, to higher ground, McCarthy said.

Patients were transported on monitors, stretchers, or wheelchairs. Others were ambulatory. Staff relocated patients in about 20 minutes. While some staff members moved patients, others grabbed what necessary medical equipment they could save. Some employees unplugged computers and other electrical devices.

Caring for patients

Meanwhile, the flooding waters did much damage to the emergency department, seeping into the walls and ruining new computer equipment that hadn't even been used. Water entered the facility, flooding the entire basement, central supply, nutrition services, medical records, and telecommunications. Damages were estimated at $1.6 million.

Emergency staffers worked together to calm and dry the patients. Meanwhile, other patients were coming into the hospital and had to be triaged from the main lobby. Caring for patients wasn't easy. The cafeteria and kitchen were flooded, so nutritional services had to work all night to provide food for staff and patients. The elevators were down, so staffers made a human chain, passing boxes of food up the stairs. Computer equipment, linens, and other equipment floated in the water. Everything that had been either ruined or contaminated by the flood was thrown out, McCarthy said.

Other problems

Repairing flood damage took a week, said Ron Kasowski, Baylor's environmental safety manager. Although the damage left the emergency department shut down for seven days, it still received patients who weren't aware that it was closed. McCarthy said the hospital had an ambulance waiting to triage patients to other facilities in the city. People with colds or minor injuries were still treated at the hospital.

Drying the emergency department wasn't an easy task. Walls had to be dried properly, soaked carpet had to be ripped out and replaced, and equipment had to be either replaced or restored. In addition, Kasowski says that his department conducted 30 separate indoor air quality tests to ensure the air was not contaminated with molds or other agents as a result of the flood.

Dealing with the media

As with most disasters, especially ones comparable to the Dallas flood, hospital staff has to deal with news crews and reporters. McCarthy said that, as a result of the flood, the hospital now trains staff members on how to compose and present themselves while talking to the media.

"It was a challenge," McCarthy said of speaking with news reporters. "You have to learn how to deal with the questions that come from reporters. We didn't want to scare the public, but [we had to] keep them informed."

Lessons learned

Baylor had disaster plans for both internal and external disasters, but still the flood took the facility by surprise. After the flood, staff members incorporated flood response into their emergency preparedness plans.

The medical center also set up a command center to improve communications within the hospital in the event of another disaster. The center features an emergency communication system, additional phone lines, and emergency checklists.

In addition, staff members also did the following:

- Worked with Dallas officials to improve drainage on the road leading to Baylor.
- Purchased six additional water pumps. The pumps, originally stored on the sixth floor, were moved to a more accessible area in the facility.
- Stored all supplies at least two feet off the ground.
- Increased staff education on dealing with internal disasters.
- Developed a bed availability matrix to help nursing staff make relocating decisions when necessary.
- Set up a phone line with the ability to place recorded messages on bed availability, elevator and utility status, food service, and other emergency information.
- Stocked up on sandbags.

While the flood may have happened five years ago, Charles Dorrell, Baylor's director of engineering, says he'll never forget the incident that greatly affected the hospital.

"I can still see the high water marks outside of the building," says Dorrell. "It serves as a reminder."

Boston facility loses records in flood

In 1999, a devastating flood dumped more than seven feet of water on a Boston nursing home, forcing the evacuation of 145 patients and destroying almost every computer and medical record in the building. Susan Redd, RN, CRRN, assistant director of nurses at Star of David Nursing Rehab and Alzheimer's Center, says losing nearly every patient record—including Medicaid cards, Minimum Data Sets (MDSs), and billing information—still affects the facility.

The facility's billing office was completely destroyed, along with the bookkeeper's office, laundry room, conference room, employee break room, and computer room. The offices of the facility administrator and director of nursing were also ruined. In all, hundreds of records were destroyed. Worse yet, there was no backup.

"We lost everything that makes the building function," says Redd.

And that was only the beginning. There was no telephone or power service, and the facility van was submerged, along with the emergency generator. Then six months later, the facility was surveyed.

"It was more difficult than usual," Redd says. "They wanted to see 18 months worth of MDSs, and we couldn't produce them. They cut us slack to a certain extent because of the flood, but think about it: You're the state, you want information, and you keep hearing, 'That was lost in the flood.' "

It was a tough way to learn the value of keeping records safe, but it did lead to changes. These days, records are regularly hauled away and stored in a secure, dry place. Also, computer records are backed up daily.

To help your facility—and your medical records—survive disaster, Redd and Mona Liblanc, MDS automation projects coordinator for the Commonwealth of Massachusetts, give the following advice:

1. **Be prepared for the worst.** "You know that disaster plan book that just gets dusty? Read it," Redd says. "I cannot express enough how everybody needs to be disaster plan-friendly. You think it won't happen to you, but when it does, you need to provide for these patients. You need to keep them safe."

2. **Do not keep all your administrative offices or records in the same place.** Star of David made that mistake and lost everything. These days the administrative offices are on different floors and different sections of the building.

3. **Anything that you cannot afford to lose should be in a safe, out-of-the-way place,** but not the basement, since it could flood. Redd also warns to be wary of windows. "You never know if something will come crashing through a window," she says.

4. **Move backup data to a secure location each month.** Liblanc recommends swapping storage space with a neighboring skilled nursing facility, or bringing the tapes and disks to your own home. Don't worry

about another facility reading your private records, because they're encrypted, Liblanc says. The backup materials should never be destroyed.

5. **Don't wait for your maintenance staff to move records to off-site storage.** Star of David now pays a company to come and pick up the records. Although they always had off-site storage, maintenance workers were in charge of moving them off-site. When maintenance workers were busy, the boxes piled up. It's worth the extra money to keep records safe, Redd says.

6. **Keep a copy of your software off-site as well.** If you need to upload software because yours crashed, you'll be able to. Keep a copy of the CD-ROM or disk somewhere safe—just in case.

7. **Create backups of MDS data on a floppy disk or tape drive.** Each day, backup data should be collected and stored. Then, at the end of the week, it should be stored in a locked, fireproof safe on another floor.

Chapter Five

Infant Abductions

Tips for staying safe with birth announcements

The JCAHO's recommendations on preventing infant abductions

Hospitals should discontinue sending birth announcements to newspapers as part of an overall plan to prevent infant abductions, says the Joint Commission on Accreditation of Healthcare Organizations (JCAHO).

In its *Sentinel Event Alert* on infant abductions, the JCAHO examined eight infant abductions and concluded that the root causes of these incidents included information-related factors, such as birth information published in the newspaper, a delay in notifying security officers of a possible abduction, and a lack of communication among caregivers.

Other root causes were insufficient security equipment, physical factors such as no line-of-sight to entrances and unmonitored elevators and stairs, and reluctance of staff members to confront unidentified people in the hospital.

What you should do

In its environment of care (EC) standards, the JCAHO expects you to address baby security through EC.1.2, which requires that hospitals plan for a secure environment.

The Joint Commission recommends the following steps:

- Discontinue publication of birth announcements in local papers
- Increase education for parents about abduction risks and their responsibility for reducing this threat
- Attach identical numbered bands to the baby, mother, and father immediately after birth
- Footprint the baby, take a color photo of the child, and record the infant's physical examination within two hours of birth
- Require maternity and other relevant staff to wear up-to-date, conspicuous identification badges with color photos
- Consider swipe-card or keypad entry options into a nursery and an infant abduction alarm system

The NCMEC's recommendations on preventing infant abductions

In its handbook *Guidelines on Prevention of and Response to Infant Abductions,* the National Center for Missing and Exploited Children (NCMEC) has the following suggestions for hospitals that choose to release birth announcement information.

For print media

- Make sure birth announcement releases do not contain home addresses or other unique information that would put the infant or the family in jeopardy after discharge
- Make sure the parents understand the risk involved with using yard signs at their homes to publicize births

For Web-based nurseries

- Internet birth announcements should contain only the fist name and last initial of the baby and parents and should not contain any references to the baby's home address
- Don't post any information until the mother and baby have been discharged and full written consent has been given
- Web sites that provide information other than the baby's first name and last initial should be password-protected so that only family members and friends can access the site
- Hospitals should remove Web photos of babies after a short time, recommends Cathy Nahirny of NCMEC

Infant abduction in Lakewood, WA

At St. Clare Hospital in Lakewood, WA, new moms are instructed to hand over their children only to hospital personnel wearing special pink tags. Security is instructed about procedures for escorting people visiting the hospital after hours, and video cameras monitor hallways and exits to the building.

Nevertheless, on August 23, 1997, an infant was abducted. A woman came to the emergency department late at night and identified herself as a medical officer from a nearby military hospital. Using a lab coat as a disguise, she gave a convincing story about being called by a patient to visit. The hospital security guard was busy with another problem, and the woman was allowed to go unescorted into the hospital. The woman talked a new mother into handing over her infant, claiming she was from the nursery. She scooted out of the building, being careful to use hallways that were the least monitored. By the time nursery staff learned of the baby's disappearance, the woman was gone.

Be decisive

When the staff discovered the abduction and telephoned quality/risk manager Marty Murray, RN, BSN, CPHQ, at home at 3:00 a.m., they interrupted the last peaceful moments of sleep she would get for a while.

Murray, relaying the story of the infant abduction during an April telephone conference of the American Society for Healthcare Risk Management, offered tips on handling an infant abduction and performing a root-cause analysis of the event.

From the moment the hospital became aware of the abduction, she says, St. Clare established a command center, developed a strategy for dealing with the media, arranged for staff emotional support, established a liaison to the family, and braced for the arrival of surveyors.

The decisions the hospital made helped to immediately affect the outcome of the case.

Dealing with the media

At the outset, the hospital decided it would take an open stance with the media. A media room was established (far away from patient care areas, where it would have been disruptive).

A media liaison was appointed. This person did not speak for the hospital, but helped arrange details such as providing refreshments, scheduling briefings, and generally telling reporters when they would have information and where they could and could not go.

As soon as possible, the media were given a description of the abductor. Sharing the details of an emergency may not always be the best course, and Murray advises hospitals to evaluate their own situation carefully, but in this case it actually helped track down the baby quickly. Acting on tips from the public, the abductor was captured, and the baby was reunited with the mother less than 24 hours after the kidnapping.

"Ninety-nine percent of the media were kind and helpful," she says. "In fact, their cooperation helped get the baby back."

Establishing a command center

An incident response team needs to be assembled immediately. Then, those people need a command center in which to work. Telephones and computers for the command center need to be dedicated solely to that purpose. Large and small tables should be available so groups of varying sizes can meet at the same time.

Secretarial support needs to be provided to the group assigned to the command center, since organization will be important. Telephone and pager numbers should be collected centrally for all people you will need to reach, both inside the hospital and outsiders such as media and police. Finally, don't forget the necessities of food, a sink, and bathroom access for the command center, since people will be spending long hours there.

Emotional support

Anticipate and brace for strong, emotional reactions from the staff. Losing an infant is disturbing, perhaps even more than you realize. The family that lost the baby will naturally need support, as will the staff.

Although most hospitals have counselors and clergy available, it's worthwhile to notify them as soon as possible so they can come around to talk with staff. Bringing them onto the scene immediately will help people deal with the stress of the event.

Anticipate surveyor interest

Both the state and the JCAHO will take an interest in the incident, and surveyors may show up at your door. In any case, they will want to review your records of your response to the event, so from the beginning, record your decisions and have the records ready.

Policies and procedures should also be readied, as the hospital will face the job of both defending existing policies and being open to suggestions for improvements.

Performing root-cause analysis

Start root-cause analysis as soon as possible to satisfy JCAHO. At St. Clare, it was underway within 48 hours of the abduction. Root-cause analysis identifies all contributing causes to the incident and tries to establish an action plan to correct and strengthen policies and procedures to prevent the abduction from recurring.

The root-cause analysis will require daily meetings at first, gradually phasing into weekly and monthly meetings as work draws to a close. At each meeting, the committee performing the analysis will look for all possible causes of the event, moving into contributing causes.

Infant abduction in Maywood, IL

Tragedy struck the Loyola University Medical Center in Maywood, IL, on May 1, 2000, when a baby boy was kidnapped from the center's nursery and later died. Loyola officials blamed a set of double doors that failed to close and lock after a sensor attached to the boy's ankle set off a security alarm.

While security equipment may be expensive and brings added protection, the Loyola incident is a sad example that such equipment isn't foolproof. So it is important that other steps be taken to prevent infants from being abducted, said Fredrick Roll, executive vice president of Health Care Security Services of Denver, CO.

According to Roll, the Loyola incident the first time that a baby abducted from a healthcare facility died at the hands of its kidnapper. The incident came on the heels of another infant abduction that occurred April 8, 2000, at SUNY Science System in Brooklyn, NY. Both events followed a 17-month period in which there were no infant abductions from healthcare facilities in the United States, according to the NCMEC. Now, Loyola faces a lawsuit from the infant's family. Although Roll did not investigate Loyola's incident, he is an expert in healthcare security, including infant abductions. He says it appears that Loyola went above and beyond what's considered essential security measures by the NCMEC.

"Electronic bracelet devices are recommended but not considered essential. What that tells me is that Loyola went over and above the minimal essentials. That was good," Roll says. "The equipment wasn't working correctly to its fullest specifications. That's a problem."

Essential guidelines

The NCMEC recently updated its list of essential and recommended measures. Essential physical security guidelines include the following:

- Every healthcare organization must develop a written assessment of the risk potential for an infant abduction.
- Install alarms, preferably with time-delay locks, on all stairwell and exit doors leading to/from or in close proximity to the maternity, nursery, neonatal and intensive care, and pediatrics units.
- All nursery doors must have self-closing hardware and must remain locked at all times. Staff members should be present at all times when an infant is in the nursery.
- Install a security camera system (using time-lapse loop tape such as those employed in banks) or digital-recording technology to monitor activity in the halls of the maternity and pediatric floors. The cameras should be placed in strategic spots in the unit to cover the nursery, hallway, stairwells, and elevators, and adjusted at an angle to capture an abductor's full face.

Testing your system

If a facility has an electronic security system in place, it is important to test it regularly. Roll says testing it at least once a day, if not every shift, is a good idea. It may be time-consuming, but staff members will know that the system is working.

According to federal investigators, one of the security lapses at Loyola was that the medical center had no specific schedule for testing the alarm system. "The hospital failed to ensure that systems designed to ensure the safety of patients in the newborn nursery were tested, functioning adequately, and implemented in the event of the abduction of an infant," the Centers for Medicare and Medicaid Services (CMS) report said.

Loyola officials would not comment on the incident other than what they reported in statements released to the press. Loyola's nursery security system was working when it was last tested nine days before the abduction, according to Loyola officials. However, an investigation revealed that there was a wiring glitch that prevented a security door outside the nursery from shutting the day of the abduction.

Always answer alarms

Meanwhile, a former Loyola nurse claims that false alarms in the maternity ward were common, resulting in staff responding to alarms with less urgency, the *Chicago Sun-Times* reported.

If what the nurse said is true, that's a serious problem, according to Roll. If your facility repeatedly has false alarms, you should find out what's causing the alarms and fix the problem or get rid of the system. An alarm is useless if people ignore it, Roll says.

According to Roll, there was a problem of repeated false alarms in one of his client hospitals. "They were having so many false alarms that people weren't paying attention to it anymore," Roll says.

Alarms are also effective only if they can be heard. Loyola's security alarm could be heard at the visitor check-in, but not in the nursery. Staff members at the check-in are required to alert nursery staff.

Staff are the core of the program

Staff members need to know they have to respond every time an alarm goes off, just in case it is an actual emergency, Roll comments.

"Electronic components are good, but they're an augmentation to your security program. The core goes to people," Roll says. "If the people are not trained, are not competent, and do not understand their role in the security operation, then you're going to have a problem." Also, it shouldn't necessarily be just security officers who respond. Nurses and other staff on the floor should be answering the call, Roll suggests.

Loyola officials said that their staff responded immediately to the alarm on May 1, 2000. Staff members did an initial count of the infants, but did not find one to be missing. A second count determined that there was a missing infant.

While medical staff may have responded quickly to the alarm, they failed to notify police immediately of the abduction, according to published reports that said Loyola didn't notify police until 56 minutes after the incident.

Restricting access to the nursery

Some hospitals, including Loyola, have gone as far as restricting access to the nursery unit. In those cases, hospital policy allows only people who are authorized or given permission by family members to be in the unit. But in Loyola's case, that policy didn't help.

The person accused of taking the 13-day-old baby from Loyola's nursery had access to the nursery because she was taking care of her newborn nephew. She was approved by the nephew's 14-year-old mother. At least one registered nurse was in the nursery during her visits, according to Loyola officials. The suspect was never observed violating any of the hospital's policies, including having contact only with her nephew, according to Loyola officials.

Other equipment and steps

If a hospital employs an electronic security system, it's also a good idea to use a video camera to capture what the abductor looks like to help hospital officials and police track down the person. Roll suggests placing the camera where it can get a good shot of the abductor's face, such as an entryway or exit to the nursery. Some hospitals have gone as far as requiring a parent or family member to always be with the infant, Roll adds.

CMS ends threat to pull funds

CMS has determined that Loyola has fixed security lapses, and the administration has rescinded its threat to cut off Medicare funding. According to CMS, a May 23 inspection showed that the security system that malfunctioned the night of the abduction is now properly working.

According to the *Chicago Sun-Times*, CMS found deficiencies "so serious they constitute an immediate threat to the health and safety of patients." CMS would not disclose exactly what those deficiencies were. Loyola took quick action to address CMS's concerns.

JCAHO steps in

JCAHO made a "special announced" survey at the center following the abduction. The hospital's accreditation status could be altered at any time, according to JCAHO.

The Joint Commission mandates what is security-sensitive. In most, if not all, cases, a nursery unit is considered a security-sensitive area. That means a hospital with a nursery must have an access control policy for the unit—whom will be allowed to have access to the unit and when should they have access?

Make sure you also have a trained critical incident response team in place. Your staff needs to know who should respond to an emergency, when they should respond, and what they should do, Roll says.

JCAHO recommendations

In 1999, JCAHO issued a sentinel event alert on infant abductions after reviewing eight hospital cases. Problems include security system breakdown, not giving staff enough education on preventing abductions, not educating patients, not monitoring elevators and stairwells, and delaying notification of security when an abduction is suspected.

JCAHO recommends requiring staff to wear security badges, controlling access to the nursery, developing prevention and emergency plans, and providing information on visitors at staff orientation.

Profile of an abductor

The NCMEC says that, in most infant abductions, the abductor is an overweight female who is driven to get an infant. Sometimes the abductor wants to replace a baby she lost or is unable to conceive or carry to term.

The offender, who generally does not have a criminal record, often visits the nursery and maternity unit several days before stealing a baby. She makes herself known to hospital personnel and becomes familiar with the infant's parents and the hospital's procedures. She repeatedly will ask detailed questions about healthcare facility procedures and the layout of the maternity unit.

The abductor often presents herself as a nurse to the victim's parents.

Crying over how to prevent infant abductions? Here's help...

A woman disguised in a lab coat came to the emergency department of a Northwest hospital one night in 1997, identifying herself as a medical officer from a nearby military hospital. She gave a convincing story about having been called by a patient to visit.

The hospital security guard, busy dealing with another problem, let the woman walk into the hospital unescorted. The woman then approached a mother with a newborn. Claiming she was from the hospital nursery, the woman talked the mother into giving her the infant. She escaped the building using hallways that were least monitored.

More than 100 infants have been reported abducted from healthcare facilities since 1985. Some babies, like the one at the Northwest hospital, have been taken right from their mothers' hospital rooms. Others were taken from newborn nurseries.

The number of infant abductions has prompted JCAHO to release a sentinel event alert regarding prevention.

Education is the best defense

Having an educated and prepared staff is the best way to prevent infant abductions, according to Fredrick Roll, executive vice president of Health Care Security Services of Denver, CO. Conducting abduction drills is one of the best ways to educate, he says.

"The number one thing that has allowed us to reduce infant abductions over the past several years is staff education," Roll says. "Drills identify weaknesses and opportunities for improvement."

The best drill is one that is practical and as close to reality as possible. Oftentimes, hospital staff will have the mock kidnapper steal a baby doll from the nursery and then begin the drill, watching all exits and searching for the infant.

Protocols for healthcare facilities may differ depending on the size of the staff and the number of beds to the facility, says Roll. Staff members should follow protocols listed by their facilities.

Once the drill has been completed, hospital staff should assess the outcome, run through a checklist to ensure that the facility's reaction was effective, and use the critique to measure response.

Exits and stairwells

Staff members of a Northeast hospital learned to control the facility's exits. The center recently installed an access control system in the likely event that a child would already be out of the facility by the time the emergency is called.

Before a drill in 1998 at a Southern hospital, staff members were instructed to be aware of everyone in their area who could be a potential abductor and to think about what to do if they spotted someone suspicious. After the drill, the staff learned the importance of having employees in each area watch elevators, exits, and stairwells.

NCMEC in Arlington, VA, offers healthcare facilities a comprehensive checklist of important measures to take to prevent abductions. Cathy Nahirny, senior analyst for the support division of the NCMEC, also recommends conducting abduction drills to complement the center's list of measures.

"You won't know if policies and protocols are going to work unless you drill, you test yourself," she says.

Announced or unannounced drills?

Should you announce when drills will occur or conduct them spontaneously? Which is more effective?

Roll believes that doing both is best. The first drill should be announced about two weeks ahead of time. Conducting an announced drill will coax staff to study the facility's procedures and protocols. A second drill should be unannounced, to make it more realistic, Roll says.

However, some security staff don't like to hold unannounced drills; they contend it unnecessarily worries parents and staff members at the hospital. At one facility, a staff member running down the stairs was so shaken up that she hurt her back, and a physician running to the parking lot almost ran into several visitors.

Roll realizes that an unannounced drill may cause some panic. He encourages staff to bring babies to their parents, so that each mother is holding her infant while the drill is conducted. Then none of the mothers will worry that it is her baby who is missing.

Drill twice each year

Roll recommends that facilities conduct at least two drills a year—one announced and one unannounced. Sometimes, a third drill should be conducted; for example, if an announced day shift drill is held, an unannounced night shift exercise should follow a couple of days later. Parent education, as well as staff education, is important. More than half of the infants stolen are taken from the mother's room, says Roll. "Most babies are given to the perpetrator by the parent."

Most abductors are female with a compulsive personality and an involvement with a significant other, says Roll. The abductor often fakes a pregnancy and is often familiar with the facility. The abductor usually investigates a number of facilities before choosing one in which to commit the crime.

Parent education

Prenatal instructors should discuss security with parents in prenatal classes, and nurses should discuss it after childbirth. Have parents sign a piece of paper acknowledging that security measures were taught, or place a poster in the room listing hospital protocol.

Tell parents to be on the lookout for suspicious people who may enter their hospital room. Nurses without proper tags should be reported.

Since JCAHO began tracking sentinel events in 1997, the Accreditation Committee of the Joint Commission's Board of Commissioners has reviewed eight cases of infant abductions. All of the abductions happened in hospitals with more than 400 beds. Five of the events occurred in the mother's room; two took place in the newborn nursery; and one happened in the neonatal intensive care unit.

In the JCAHO Environment of Care, Security-Related Standards, "security-sensitive" areas, such as areas with infants, are asked to have an access control plan, says Roll. Such areas may feature anything from signs that read "Authorized personnel only" to sophisticated electrical devices.

"Providing safety and security measures to minimize the potential of an infant abduction should be the responsibility of all healthcare staff members," Roll says.

"Protocols must be developed based upon the vulnerabilities identified as part of the assessment process. A team approach to this problem is one of the best methods of prevention," he continues.

Chapter Six

Shootings

Columbine shooting tests emergency response plan

What measures should the emergency department use to decide when an influx of patients constitutes a problem serious enough to trigger a hospital's emergency response plan? That's one of the questions lingering at Littleton (CO) Adventist Hospital following the student shootings at Columbine High School in 1999.

Kelli Dahl, environmental health and safety manager for Porter and Littleton Adventist hospitals, says that in the wake of the shootings that drew national attention to the Denver suburb, the 132-bed Littleton hospital has been looking closely at its emergency response plan. While the hospital did not handle the most critical patients from the shootings, it did handle the highest number of shooting victims, and the incident provided some valuable lessons for polishing the hospital's disaster response plan.

The value of drills

In general, Dahl credits hospital staff with an excellent response to the influx of 10 patients, grieving family, hordes of media, and an unexpected number of community volunteers who wanted to help in the tragedy. A disaster drill, which included mock victims from a fake school bus accident just five days before the shooting, helped prepare staff for the crisis.

"It was just the first time that I as a safety officer held drills with mass casualty patients," Dahl says, "and as redundant as they seem, I'll do them every year."

Still, Dahl says, there are lessons the Columbine shooting taught that disaster drills cannot teach.

Early warning

One of the biggest issues that cropped up in this incident was establishing a protocol for deciding when to activate the hospital's emergency response plan. Although rumors were popping for hours about the crisis at the school, details were hard to come by. Dahl, who was stationed at Littleton's sister hospital, was not aware of the high school tragedy unfolding.

Meanwhile, the emergency department director assessed the situation first from a purely clinical point of view. The hospital had enough beds, and it could handle the patients in the emergency department, so it wasn't immediately obvious that the emergency response plan needed to be activated.

So by the time the plan was activated and Dahl and other officials received the page signaling them to establish the incident command post, patients and the media were already at the hospital. This delay prompted complaints that the command post phones weren't answered in the early stages of the incident. In turn, this prompted some confusion later on about whether the command post was up and running.

In the future, Dahl says, the emergency department will establish a protocol for deciding what warrants activation of the plan. It may include such things as the number of patients expected, anticipated media response, and consultation with others involved in emergency response planning. Also, the hospital may add an early notification system to the plan, so that if it seems there's a chance that the plan will have to be activated, some key personnel will be notified.

Dealing with the media

A second issue the facility will address in future drills is more careful planning for media access. While the facility's disaster plan calls for a media room to be established—where press members are to be held and given updates—it was not put into place in the early stages of the event. It was only when a hospital vice president saw that television cameras had the ability to film patients being brought into the emergency department and families in the halls that the media room rules were invoked.

"That's something we will definitely address," Dahl says.

While security at the perimeter of the hospital grounds was adequate, the media needed more clear direction about where they could and could not go. The new plan for media will balance the need for flexibility with the need for privacy.

Volunteer overload

Not only was the media overwhelming, but the hospital was also flooded by people who were touched by the tragedy and wanted to help. While the emergency department focused on treating patients, it soon became clear that the problem in the emergency department was too many helping hands rather than too few. Volunteers should have been referred to the personnel pool, where they could be assigned a duty or sent home with a polite "No thanks," says Dahl.

Personnel pool

In this case, grief counselors who were not affiliated with the hospital volunteered their services and had to be told gently but firmly that they were not needed. The personnel pool would have been the appropriate place to interview potential volunteers, rather than leaving that chore to the harried ED staff.

Again, Dahl stresses, this points to the need to have the personnel pool up and running as soon as possible, and to educate everyone—volunteers, family, media, and staff—that the place to go first is the command post, and from there they will be routed to wherever they are needed.

Do not shut down early

Another important lesson the hospital learned was not to shut down the command post too soon. Initially, the command post operated for six hours, and then shut down after the first rush of patients and family subsided. But during the following shift, 60 phone calls came in from people looking for information. The media were following up on stories, families were trying to track down relatives, and volunteers were calling to offer services. In retrospect, Dahl says, she wishes the command post had stayed open longer.

Refinements planned

The hospital plans to follow up the incident with some refinements to its emergency response plan, but in general, Dahl notes that the facility is pleased with the way it handled the incident.

Columbine shooting analysis points to need for disaster planning

Analysis of hospital emergency preparedness during 1999's Columbine High School shootings in Colorado highlights the need for healthcare facilities to learn the incident command system (ICS), and the starting point is with leaders in your medical center. That advice comes from a doctor who treated some of the wounded students from the shooting and who has since examined how hospitals and emergency services responded to the incident.

"Get your key people, your leaders, involved [with the ICS and disaster drilling] . . . Otherwise, you then have personnel under them who won't take it seriously," says Michael Hunt, MD, the EMS medical director at Swedish Medical Center in Englewood, CO. Hunt spoke at the NFPA's recent World Fire Safety Congress in Denver.

Disaster preparedness

The ICS is a disaster planning model that sets up a structured emergency response to help coordinate decision-making among various emergency services. NFPA 99, Healthcare Facilities, outlines the steps to setting up an ICS.

The belief in the industry is that the Joint Commission on Accreditation of Healthcare Organizations (JCAHO) will eventually require healthcare facilities to use the ICS as part of its environment of care standards. The JCAHO already requires hospitals to conduct two disaster drills each year.

Hunt supports the idea of practicing specific disaster scenarios during those drills. As part of that training, healthcare sites should be ready for potential chemical and biological weapon use. He says that field data suggest that, when people are exposed to chemicals during disasters, fewer than 20% get decontaminated at the scene, which means they show up at the hospital as hazardous threats. If health workers aren't careful in handling these patients, they can contaminate the emergency room, and at that point, you've merely relocated the exposure problem into the hospital, Hunt says.

Chemical weapon knowledge

Hunt admits that he did not consider this scenario when treating some of the Columbine victims, even though it later came out that the suspects were familiar with chemical bombs.

"I was thinking about kids with bullet holes in them," Hunt recalls. "It wasn't until three days later that I wondered if these [suspects] had any [knowledge] about chemical weapons."

While it would be impossible to predict a high school shooting such as the one in Colorado, Hunt suggests that you look around your community for potential disasters. For example, do you have an airport in your region? Does your city have a water supply susceptible to terrorism?

Other suggestions

Some other advice from Hunt on the hospital end of disaster planning includes the following:

- Push for a coordinated communication system among all agencies and sites that will aid in a disaster response. A problem with the Columbine response was that authorities did not talk to each other on a dedicated channel, which created problems getting the correct information out to everyone, Hunt says.
- Decide ahead of time whether physicians should go to the scene of a disaster or remain in the hospital waiting for victims.
- Use triage tags at the scene to identify victims so that hospital personnel know whom they're treating when victims arrive at the hospital.
- Following a disaster, critique the hospital's response, and look for things that went wrong and how other actions could have been better. Use this critique to enhance future disaster drills and ICS training.

Offer "incident stress debriefing" to your staff members and let them stay in touch with their own families during the disaster. "I probably made my biggest mistake [during the Columbine response] by not calling my wife," Hunt says. "She knew I was out there, but I never called her. She didn't know what was going on."

Armed or unarmed security officers?

Should security officers at your facility be armed? It's a question every hospital faces.

Before making this decision, you should consider a number of things, according to Kevin A. Dumdai, safety/security supervisor at North Dakota State Hospital, and Thomas Huser, health and safety specialist for St. Vincent's Hospital and Healthcare Center in Indianapolis, IN. First, staff members should assess the area in which the facility is located. Is there a high crime rate or high risk, or is there a low crime rate and little risk?

"It's going to be up to the demographics," says Huser. "It's [the hospital's] individual decision–what's going to be best for their employees and their patients."

A comprehensive security/risk assessment starts with an examination of statistical information on regional and community criminal activity, Dumdai says. Second, the development of a security management plan should consider the working aspects of your present-day program, including a review of policies and procedures, facility design features, and security technologies.

Performance indicators should measure the effectiveness of the program, pointing out the strengths and weaknesses of the department. They can be further used in determining what corrective action to take when indicators show a problem. You should assess the number of weapons-related incidents that have occurred either in your hospital or in the nearby area.

Three-part protocol

St. Vincent's staff members follow three different protocols. There are armed security officers at the main campus, while there is limited access to the facility's mental health building. Security officers carry firearms on the first floor of the mental health building, but guns must be locked in safe boxes before a security officer is permitted to enter the second floor, where patients stay.

At St. Vincent's other general care facility, in Carmel, IN, security officers are not allowed to carry firearms, according to Huser. The perception is that Carmel is safer because it is further from Indianapolis. However, perception does not always match reality. Two years ago, a bank robber shot five people, killing three, only a few blocks away from the Carmel facility. The robber was then found dead in a tree on adjacent property from a self-inflicted bullet wound. And four years ago, three children were executed less than a mile from the facility.

Weapons are not allowed on the premises at North Dakota State Hospital, a state psychiatric care facility for adolescent, chemical-dependent and psychiatric patients. Security personnel are trained for their position and must also be certified in therapeutic intervention.

Meanwhile, Dumdai follows a simpler rule at North Dakota: No weapons allowed, period. Security officers dress in plain clothes to reduce patient anxiety. The officers, however, wear security badges and are equipped with two-way radios. Communication devices are interfaced with the hospital's communication system for immediate response. The interface allows officers to directly communicate with rescue personnel and 9-1-1 dispatch.

Another policy in place

At the Bay Medical Center in Panama City, FL, Paul Lockwood, manager of safety and protection services, says that his security officers are not armed, mainly because the facility conducts more than 1,500 psychiatric patient watches annually. No other persons except on-duty law enforcement are permitted to carry firearms into the facility. All entrances have signs that read "No Firearms Allowed."

The only place law enforcement officers are prohibited from carrying their weapons is the mental health unit. They must secure the sidearm in a gun locker located outside the unit.

Bay Medical has developed a detailed policy on forensic staff who may be with a patient inmate. If the inmate were to get out of control, it is the responsibility of the hospital's security officers, not the armed law enforcement officer guarding the patient, to intervene. Lockwood says that the policy was created to prevent inmates from getting close to weapons.

Public perception

Choosing whether to arm officers does not merely depend on high crime rates. It also depends on the public's opinion of whether guns are needed in healthcare facilities.

Proponents of Florida's bill fear that weapons brought into a facility could be used against employees, patients, and visitors. Should you decide to arm your security officers, be warned. Some might perceive the move as turning the facility into an armed encampment, says Huser. They might be nervous about having guns on the premises.

But, while there are those who are against weapons in a healthcare facility, others believe that security officers need to carry weapons.

Huser says that employees at his facility don't really object to security officers having weapons because people are used to the policy. Officers had firearms at their old campus before moving to the new facility, he says. But for those facilities that are switching from unarmed to armed officers, there will be questions.

"Throughout your whole staff, the question that's going to be asked is 'Why?' " Huser says. "That means staff education."

Visitors and other employees

Visitors and employees other than security officers and on-duty police officers are not allowed to carry weapons on the premises at St. Vincent's, according to Huser.

Employees are informed of the facility's policy during orientation. Visitors are not checked with a metal detector when they enter the building, but if a firearm is discovered on their person, they are asked to leave the weapon in their car or secure it in a safe box in the security office.

All incoming personnel at North Dakota are monitored via closed-circuit television, with the entrance door secured by a magnetic locking device. All admissions are searched and scanned by a metal detector, and law enforcement officers are provided with gun lockers to secure their firearms, Dumdai says.

Liability

With armed security officers comes liability, Huser warns. There are a number of things to consider before you allow officers to carry a firearm.

You have to worry about someone getting shot, drawing a firearm at an inappropriate time, or improperly threatening to use the weapon. Problems can come either from someone who manages to take the weapon away from an officer or from the officer himself.

Training

Officers hired at St. Vincent's must be deputized by the Sheriff's department as well as undergo 75 hours of orientation training at the facility. Officers also undergo weapons retention training, so they are prepared if someone tries to steal their gun from them.

"The most important thing is training, training, training," Huser says.

Scrutinizing staff

Hospitals should always be careful about whom they hire, especially when hiring an employee who has access to a firearm, Huser warns.

Before St. Vincent hires a security officer, he or she is interviewed extensively. The hospital conducts a criminal background check, and if the hospital is hiring from a private security company, staff makes sure it is a reputable company.

Cost

In addition to weighing the risks of having an armed security force, you have to consider the costs involved. The costs will be different for each facility, depending on how many officers you have as well as what types of weapons they carry. At St. Vincent's, officers are allowed to carry either a revolver or a semi-automatic gun. The officer pays for and owns the weapon. You should also consider legal costs if, for example, the weapons are not handled properly and an incident occurs.

Hospitals unprepared for violence

Know the warning signs

Hospitals should learn to recognize the warning signs and events that might trigger violence among patients or workers, since violence could erupt at any time, says Fredrick Roll, CHPA-F, CPP, executive vice president of Healthcare Security Services in Denver, CO.

"At least we need to be aware of some of the potential problems that can happen," advises Roll, a leading expert in healthcare security.

Hospitals must be aware that trouble can occur anywhere and at any time. For example, on June 28, 2000, a resident physician who had been fired from the University of Washington Medical Center allegedly shot and killed a high-ranking doctor at the center before turning the gun on himself, CNN news reported. Apparently the resident physician was told that his contract as a resident would not be renewed, harming his prospects for future employment. The incident occurred away from any patient care areas.

Furthermore, a report from the *Journal of Healthcare Safety, Compliance & Infection Control* states that healthcare workers have a high risk for being attacked on the job. But most hospitals and other healthcare providers are "flying by the seat of their pants" when it comes to making contingency plans for violence in the workplace, Roll says.

Roll says facilities should pay attention to these nine warning signs of trouble:

- Employees who threaten revenge
- Employees who have difficulty with authority
- Employees who become angry or upset easily
- Employees who act paranoid and do things such as write down in a notebook what they consider insulting comments
- Employees who do not see humor in any situation
- Employees who do not show sensitivity in any form
- Employees who openly speak of weapons in the context of "teaching people a lesson"
- Employees who often speak of violent movies or books they have seen or read
- Employees who often threaten to sue

Some employees could also resort to violence to resolve disputes with their co-workers, he adds. Other precipitating events leading to violence could include being passed over for promotion, rejection of a relationship, and discrimination. If you have to terminate a worker who is prone to violence, be aware that, on the anniversary of his or her termination date, this individual might seek revenge, Roll says.

Common risks and vulnerabilities

Roll outlines a number of vulnerabilities in healthcare facilities based on examinations of security systems in hospitals around the country. These risks include the following:

- Uncontrolled access and uncontrolled after-hours access

- Inadequate sensitive-area security programs
- Inadequate security staffing and deployment
- Inadequate security training
- Poor visitation policies and procedures
- Inadequate records and reports

Another risk is the lack of a security management plan. Having such a plan is not only important, it is a JCAHO requirement.

Preventative steps

You can take action to stop violence on the job before it happens, Roll says. Measures you can take to prevent violent actions include identifying potential risks and vulnerabilities, developing appropriate recommendations, weighing the risk against the cost of the recommendation, and implementing a plan for corrective action. (See Appendix H for tips on hazard prevention.) Your organization should also conduct assessments at your facility if there are any significant changes, such as a change in the patient mix, new construction, or any major renovations, Roll adds.

Treating patients

Healthcare workers are not only at risk of violence from co-workers, they also could be assaulted or injured by patients. Healthcare workers face the prevalence of handguns and other weapons in society in their care of disturbed and violent individuals, mentally ill patients, gang members, drug and alcohol abusers, and those who are frustrated by long waits in the emergency department. When putting a security management plan together, you should assess the area in which your facility is located as well as the area's demographics, Rolls advises. Is your facility in a high crime area? What crimes are prevalent and could filter into your building?

Written prevention program

In creating a written violence prevention program, it is important to do a work site analysis, Roll says. Establish an assessment team to examine the potential for workplace violence and determine the appropriate preventative action. The analysis should include examining employee tasks and identifying hazards, conditions, operations, and situations that could lead to violence.

Evaluate existing security systems and review injury and illness records and workers' compensation claims to identify patterns of assaults, Roll suggests. Roll also suggests developing screening surveys to encourage comments from employees on what security improvements need to be made.

OSHA guidelines

Facilities should also be aware that OSHA has outlined some guidelines for preventing violence against healthcare workers. Also known as OSHA #3148, the guidelines are intended to assist employers in creating violence prevention programs. Although the guidelines are not standards or regulations, they do offer some good assistance. The guidelines are performance-based and stress that there should be "zero tolerance" for violence. According to the guidelines, employers should also recognize that violence may come from many different sources.

Although the guidelines are not a requirement, OSHA may still cite and fine a facility under its "General Duty Clause" for not providing a safe working environment for its employees.

Chapter Seven

Nature's Wrath

Earthquake tests the disaster plans of Seattle hospitals

Keep talking

Following a 6.8 magnitude earthquake in February 2001, some employees at Western State Hospital in Steilacoom, WA, left with little warning to check on their homes and families. Many returned to assist once they were satisfied that their loved ones were safe, says Kris Flowers, the facility's public information coordinator.

However, to ensure that patient care and security needs were met, Western State detained remaining employees once administrators found out some had left—and it was not a popular decision.

"For staff morale, [detaining people] is not a good thing to do," Flowers says. Now, the hospital is coming up with a new emergency management policy that balances worker worries during a disaster with the need to keep them on the job during a critical period.

Those in charge are leaning toward the idea of temporarily letting non-patient care employees leave the workplace, perhaps for a couple of hours, before requiring them to return, she adds. Also, the hospital is considering an arrangement with a sister facility in Eastern Washington to act as a remote liaison office between family members and employees who are unable talk on overburdened local phone lines.

Staff members are being asked to set up their own personal arrangements with a contact person outside their local area, says Irvin Warner, facilities director at Western State.

Bringing people in

After an earthquake, call in extra safety and plant staff members and have them available 24 hours a day, because things will continue to break, says Duane Mariotti, director of clinical engineering and acting director of facility engineering at Harborview Medical Center in Seattle. Also, find a structural engineer quickly, because you'll need someone to certify that a building is safe following a quake, Mariotti says.

Harborview sustained cracks up to five inches wide in places between the new and older wings of the main hospital, but greater damage occurred in an outpatient clinic. Luckily, hospital safety crews quickly inspected the latter building, Mariotti says. Facility directors and safety officers should determine ahead of time who will check off-campus sites, he suggests.

Over at Western State, the facility plans to develop a personnel pool so that, in the future, a system is in place to call in more workers when a disaster plan is in effect. On the day of the quake, many off-duty employees came in just in case they were needed.

Complicated evacuations

Evacuations were not easy at Western State following the quake. The hospital decided to evacuate 2,500 patients and employees—and in some cases, it may have been a hasty choice.

"I think one of the mistakes we made, based on critiques we got, was we began to evacuate patients before we were sure they had to be evacuated," Flowers says. In a lot of respects, the evacuations were based on gut reactions following the trembling.

For example, the hospital began evacuating some patients without first waiting to see if the building they were in was damaged enough to abandon, she says. A quick risk assessment—comparing building damage against the health risks to patients—might have prevented unneeded evacuations, she adds.

Adding to the problems is that Western State houses psychiatric and geriatric patients, as well as court-committed individuals, so security is always an issue, even without an earthquake.

High-risk patients

One entire building deemed unusable contained 239 high-risk patients whom staff members had to relocate to a fenced-in area outside the building in the immediate moments after the quake. The hospital put some of these patients in a bus until enough extra employees could be called in to provide adequate coverage, Warner says.

Eventually, workers brought 30 patients who were being held pending court appearances to an unoccupied locked ward, while the rest of the high-risk patients spent the night in a hospital gymnasium under tight security.

Workplace violence is a concern, and staff members didn't want things to get out of control following the quake. "Those who were here under the state's criminal commitment law had adequate security," Flowers says.

Know your locals

The hospital focused on maintaining peace and quiet following the earthquake, she says. At the incident command center, it was well known what the risks were from the patients. Relief also came from the local police department and sheriff's office, which sent about 20 people to the hospital within an hour of the quake to help out. Firefighters and municipal building inspectors also came to the scene.

The authorities knew about the dangers of unsecured patients at Western State based on prior discussions and sitdowns with hospital administrators, Flowers says. She emphasizes how important it is for all hospitals to talk to fire and police officials so that they know what your facility does and the risks involved.

Had Western State not gotten to know public safety officials beforehand, Flowers says they may not have thought to provide extra help that day. In the following days, the police worked with the hospital to safely transfer the patients to new, secure areas.

Interestingly enough, all the patients behaved well following the earthquake. There are typically 20–25 aggressive incidents each day, including assaults, at the facility, but on the day of the quake, there were none, Flowers says. Some patients even helped comfort fellow patients and distribute food and blankets to others, she adds.

Communications problems

In examining your communication strategies, think about how staff members will talk to each other and people in the community if a quake or other emergency strikes.

"The [phone] lines were so busy here that nobody could call through" after the tremor, says Irvin Warner. Local calls in the area of the quake were very difficult to make, though long-distance calls got through.

Cell phone letdown

Very few cell phone connections could be made either, because the load on the cellular system exceeded its capabilities, says Flowers.

In the aftermath of the quake, Western State plans to revise its disaster plan to designate people as "runners"—essentially, staff members who will traverse the hospital's units and buildings if the phone lines don't work during an incident.

It is ironic to think that technology would take a seat behind old-fashioned legwork, but in some cases messengers scuttling among the property may be more reliable than phones during a disaster response and recovery, Flowers adds.

Test your policies

Regularly test any community-based radio systems your hospital might be a part of, says Mariotti.

After the quake, a county radio system the hospital was part of "failed miserably" because it was overloaded, Mariotti says. He suggests facilities install a campus-wide public address system so announcements can be made to many buildings and all staff members at one time, which comes in handy if regular phone lines go down.

You should also conduct emergency drills with failed communication scenarios. "Do them, because you really learn," Mariotti says.

Accepting patients?

Some hospitals must also prepare for a unique role if a major earthquake hits: dealing with any structural damage while throngs of people possibly show up with injuries. Harborview continued to accept trauma patients who arrived with earthquake-related wounds while engineers surveyed the facility's damage.

"Nobody ever talks about that side of hospital work," says Mariotti. "We get about 15 minutes to make sure our building's okay, and then have to prepare to take care of the patients."

This balancing act can become even trickier if your healthcare facility is a designated triage center in a community or county disaster plan, so make sure you have provisions in place for how to deal simultaneously with the responsibilities of treating patients and assessing structural problems.

Wintertime problems: Try a little warmth and preparedness

For many regions, and most of you will have to deal with related life safety problems—if you haven't already—ranging from frozen pipes to doorways blocked with snow.

Even if Old Man Winter has cooperated with you so far, it doesn't hurt to be proactive and think about how your facility might deal with potential weather problems.

"I don't think enough thought is given to 'what if this, what if that,'" says Ray Moughalian, BSIE, ASAE, president of RM Associates in Haverhill, MA, a facilities management consulting firm.

Appendix I provides a checklist for winter safety hazards. Below, we address three specific areas on the winter hazard radar: snow removal, freezing pipes, and utility problems.

Snow removal

Yes, you've heard time and again about removing snow and ice from entrances and exit doors. You've probably even had staff members and visitors complaining about snow piling up.

But things could get worse than a complaint: A former ambulance worker has sued Maine General Medical Center in Augusta, claiming she slipped on black ice and permanently injured her back while moving a patient into the emergency room entrance in 1994.

The lawsuit claims the hospital and its employees were negligent in not clearing the ice from the area and failed to warn people that it was dangerous even after maintenance staff members were alerted about the icy conditions, according to the *Kennebec Journal.* The hospital denies any wrongdoing.

Don't forget, the Joint Commission on Accreditation of Healthcare Organizations (JCAHO) can cite hospitals for not clearing walkways of ice and snow under Question 5M of the *Statement of Conditions.*

To avoid such potential problems, you should prioritize removal efforts, says Robert Westenberger, MCO, corporate director of safety and regulatory compliance at Saint Clare's Health Services in Denville, NJ. Here are three important areas Westenberger suggests that you focus on:

- Required exits and walks (also fire escapes if your building has them)
- Fire truck lanes
- Fire hydrants and other fire department connections

You must also pay particular attention to exit discharges in your hospital that are not paved to a public way because you are still responsible for making sure people can use them safely.

"Many times, they are not paved, so the snow removal is forgotten," Moughalian says. "Those things [should be] a top priority for snow removal."

Other life safety experts remind facilities that they should determine where to put plowed snow if they are in a crowded area without a lot of free space, such as a downtown hospital.

Freezing pipes

Aside from normal inspection, testing, and maintenance, you should give extra care to sprinkler pipes in areas that could be exposed to cold temperatures. Such areas commonly include attics, ceiling voids, garages, vestibules between two sets of doors, and loading docks.

"I find that overhangs and false building facades are the biggest problem," Westenberger says. "It doesn't take much to freeze standing water. Designers assume that building heat will always migrate to these areas."

He likes to look at two areas when it comes to suppression systems:

- Dry systems—You need to verify that a dry system is indeed dry; in other words, that there isn't water in it, Westenberger says. This inspection should include looking at check valves, air valves, and clapper valves.

- Wet systems—If your wet system has a glycol mixture, you should double-check the glycol percentage and also "freeze test" the mixture to find out what temperature is good for the system. Don't assume an initial reading that was acceptable will remain unchanged, because as you conduct your quarterly flow tests, you add fresh water and change your glycol mix. Also make sure you properly heat the area.

Utility problems

A fast-moving storm can immediately knock down powerlines and jeopardize water supplies, but sometimes the storm's aftermath can be just as devastating. A couple of years ago, many regions, including the Southeast and the Northeast, were without power or communications because of nasty ice storms.

"An ice storm could knock you out for a week," says Moughalian.

He adds that you shouldn't overlook the phone system when you're thinking about the loss of power or water.

"In the failure plans, they should be addressing . . . telecommunications and what happens if the phone system is down," he says.

Along with many other business customers, Sinai Samaritan Medical Center in Milwaukee lost its steam heat for about six hours on February 5, 2001. However, having experienced outages before, the hospital was prepared, says spokesperson Jennifer Gross.

Upon getting the news of the outage from the power company, Sinai Medical got extra blankets ready and also closed window blinds in areas where drafts were a concern. Many of the patient sleeping rooms are on the upper floors of the facility, so the site was able to preserve heat for a period of time in those areas.

"The largest complaint we got was maybe the hot water didn't come on as quickly as people would've liked," Gross says. "Maybe there was a few degrees' difference, but nobody was shivering."

Ice storm in Nebraska

In the fall of 1997, around most of the country, folks were visiting theaters to see the movie "The Ice Storm." In Omaha, NE, citizens just had to look out their windows to see what a real ice storm looked like. And the reality was not nearly as much fun as the movie.

Coping with sport utility vehicles (SUVs) that turned out to be useless, make-shift telephone systems, shelters that weren't supposed to be shelters, and a unique hospital-wide car pool system, the six hospitals in Omaha stayed up and running,

And, according to Peg Luebbert, MS, MT (ASCP), SC, CIC, risk management specialist at Alegent Health Systems, a lot of valuable lessons were learned. If it accomplished nothing else, at least the storm made it clear to hospital employees why they are asked to participate in so many disaster drills.

"We heard over and over again, 'So this is why the Joint Commission makes us do those drills,'" she says. "When the generator has to kick in ten times in one night, you're glad you've made sure it's working."

Treating the injured

By far, the most casualties from the storm were the trees in Omaha. Estimates say that as many as half of them were damaged. They came down across roads, roofs, electrical wires, and anything on the ground. The result was that many smaller roads were impassable and electricity was lost to some parts of the city for 10 days.

That posed a number of challenges to the hospitals. First, the emergency rooms were swamped with people seeking treatment from injuries sustained while doing everything from cutting up tree limbs to clearing driveways.

Complicating matters was the fact that many hospital employees were stranded in their homes, blocked in by trees. Alegent formed a transportation system, relying on people with four-wheel drive vehicles to ferry employees to and from work.

The hospital broke the city down into ZIP codes and geographically located each employee on one central map. Drivers were then dispatched to bring in people from all departments who lived in the same area, picking them up at spots accessible to roads and near their houses.

Ironically, several of the hospital's doctors had to be ferried from home even though they owned four-wheel drive sport utility vehicles. The problem? The SUVs were tucked snug inside their garages, with doors that need electricity to open.

At the hospital

Inside the hospitals, people faced challenges as well. And they came up with some unique solutions. In one hospital, the telephone system crashed for an extended period. Without regular phones, the hospital dispatched security officers to each floor with a walkie-talkie to relay messages from a central communications station. And each unit was assigned a cell phone to keep direct communications open.

Meanwhile, Alegent Health Midlands Community Hospital was turned into a shelter for a while, albeit somewhat by accident. The hospital was on the Red Cross list of potential shelter spots to be used if the population needing shelter expanded beyond what could be handled at primary shelters. The idea, says Nancy Noda, manager for safety and infection control, was that the hospital could open up its cafeteria, if needed, to give people a warm place to sit.

Unfortunately, word got out through the fire department that the hospital itself was open as a shelter and was a good place for people with health concerns to go. While most people were able to be routed to the regular shelters, several people with legitimate health needs were admitted for observation while their homes were without power. Noda says the incident pointed out the need to add an additional level of sheltering to the local emergency shelter program—one that would serve people in need of medical monitoring.

"We got lots of phone calls from people with chronic illness, people with electric beds, some with MS," she says. "A regular shelter isn't the place for those people."

Noda says plans to create a shelter to serve people with medical conditions are now in the works.

Tropical Storm Floyd: Power failure leads to patient death

During Tropical Storm Floyd on September 17, 1999, a scary situation resulted in a worst-case scenario for Rhode Island Hospital in Providence, RI: A power outage allegedly led to a patient's death because there was no electricity for a ventilator.

At press time, investigations are still searching for the reason the healthcare facility's generators did not work during the blackout, which occurred after a piece of debris crashed into a Narragansett Electric substation. Although Narragansett Electric restored power in eight minutes, Rhode Island Hospital was unable to accept the feed, and its own generators did not work, leaving the facility without power for nearly two hours, according to the *Providence Journal*.

Rhode Island Hospital is a 719-bed facility affiliated with Brown University's School of Medicine. There are 30 buildings on the hospital's campus. After the generator failed to turn on, crews from the Providence Fire Department responded with portable generators to help restore some power to the hospital.

Utility stands by its system

On October 1, officials from Narragansett Electric told the state's Civil Preparedness Advisory Council that the company's systems worked properly during the blackout, the *Journal* reported.

Rhode Island Hospital officials said their site does not have an independent backup generator. The hospital's own power plant is the primary source for electricity, while about one-third of the power is purchased from Narragansett Electric. The power company is the hospital's only backup, an official told the council.

The *Journal* reported that the hospital and the utility company agreed that the "sharing" system failed. The *Journal* also quoted a Narragansett engineer who said that, although the system was designed to protect against long-term power losses, those features were never tested.

NFPA requirements

NFPA 99, Health Care Facilities, requires facilities to test emergency generators every month under paragraph 3-4.4.1.1. It is not clear whether these requirements would apply to the Rhode Island Hospital situation.

Some life safety experts indicate that, while NFPA 99 doesn't specifically address a power setup such as Rhode Island Hospital's, the intent of the code seems to imply that facilities should test all backup power systems. One question that experts believe will be raised is whether the hospital provided a minimum level of care to protect patients and staff.

Russell Phillips, president of Russell Phillips & Associates in Rochester, NY, says that, in general, healthcare facilities should look at three common factors that lead to generator problems: The transfer switch fails, the generator's batteries don't work, or the generator's fuel pump malfunctions.

Staff reaction

According to the *Journal*, staff members at the hospital responded to the outage in the following ways:

- Based on emergency drill training, employees grabbed flashlights and began triage where needed
- When it was clear the ventilators weren't working, nurses grabbed oxygen bags and began manually ventilating patients
- Additional off-duty staff members were called in
- Nurses set up a system to get medicine from the basement pharmacy after the computerized medicine dispensary shut down

Is your facility ready for nature's wrath?

The tornadoes that swept through Jarrell, TX, in May 1997, killing 27 people and injuring many others, serve as a reminder of how important it is that staff know how to react when a disaster strikes. It is crucial that safety officers conduct useful drills that improve the hospital's overall readiness for an emergency situation.

Although it is easy to shrug off disasters that occur thousands of miles away, keep in mind that nearly every region of the country experienced some type of natural disaster in the 1990s: floods in the Midwest and Northeast, earthquakes and fires in the West, and hurricanes and tornadoes in the South.

By preparing for a severe weather emergency or any other event classified as a disaster, you will have a better chance of surviving it.

Stage realistic drills

For the past few years, Melissa Mitchell, safety analyst at Ochsner Medical Institutions, New Orleans, LA, has successfully conducted a week-long hurricane drill at her facility. Although the drill is now a bit tiresome, staff respond well to it because they know that it's just a matter of time before a hurricane actually hits their area. "Hurricane season here starts on June 1, and in New Orleans it's a big threat. Staff take it seriously because our number has to be coming up soon," she says.

Mitchell went to her local library to research past hurricanes in the New Orleans area and copied newspaper articles about the storm. On the first day of the drill, she sends a notice to personnel alerting them that a hurricane is in the Caribbean. Each day, she sends updates with storm coordinate information.

"As the storm comes closer, [staff] are supposed to implement plans. For example, purchasing should call vendors for extra supplies. Last year, once the hurricane hit, we staged damaged areas in the hospital. We broke windows in one wing, and staff had to find alternate places for patients," she says.

Success factors

Careful pre-planning, coordinated execution, and quick and thorough post-drill evaluation are the key ingredients to improving disaster readiness.

Pre-planning

Martha Pearce, WSO, CSM, CSSD, director of the department of protective services at Albert Einstein Healthcare Network, Philadelphia, PA, says safety officers should think about the patients they serve and then plan for the worst-case scenario.

Also, when staff say it will never happen at their facility, recount first-hand experiences of other hospitals. "Relating experiences makes it real for them," she says.

Execution

With planning and education taken care of, executing a drill is the easy part. But Doug Thyne, safety manager at North Chicago VA Medical Center, says each department must focus on the goals and objectives.

"Knowing what you need to accomplish and focusing on that during a drill is critical if the exercise is to be of any value," he says.

Evaluation and critique

Critique the disaster exercises within 24 hours after the drill. Each participant should receive a summary of the drill, with an itemized, minute-by-minute recounting.

Thyne has his group go over every problem that occurred during the drill. The committee then proposes a recommended solution, and the medical center director reviews and comments on the recommendations.

Appendices

Appendix A

Steps to take in response to a biological or chemical attack

Below you will find information from the Centers for Disease Control and Prevention's (CDC) Bioterrorism Readiness Plan: A Template for Healthcare Facilities. The complete report can be found at *www.healthsafetyinfo.com/pdf/bioterrorism.pdf*.

1. Healthcare facilities may be the initial site of recognition and response to bioterrorism events. If a bioterrorism event is suspected, local emergency response systems should be activated, including local infection control personnel, the healthcare facility administration, local and state health departments, the FBI field office, the CDC, the police, and medical emergency services.

2. It is important to identify the agent used in the attack. Symptoms, as well as laboratory confirmation, are helpful in determining the possibility of a bioterrorism-related outbreak. Symptoms of a possible outbreak include the following:

- A rapidly increasing disease incidence in a normally healthy population
- An unusual increase in the number of people seeking care, especially with fever, respiratory, or gastrointestinal complaints
- Clusters of patients arriving from a single locale
- Lower attack rates among people who had been indoors
- Any patient presenting with a disease that is relatively uncommon and has bioterrorism potential such as pulmonary anthrax, tularemia, or plague

3. All patients who are suspected of being infected should be managed using standard precautions, which include hand washing, gloves, mask/eye protection or face shields, and gowns.

4. Each facility should have procedures for the routine care, cleaning, and disinfection of equipment and surfaces. Germicidal cleaning agents should be available in patient care areas. Reusable equipment should not be used for another patient until properly cleaned and reprocessed. Patient linen should be properly cared for, and contaminated waste should be handled in accordance with federal, state, and local laws.

5. When developing a bioterrorism response plan, facilities should consider available locations and procedures for patient decontamination prior to facility entry.

6. Local and state health departments should be consulted when determining whether to decontaminate a patient. If decontamination is necessary, clothing may have to be removed and properly disposed of. Bathing patients with bleach solutions or other potentially harmful practices should be avoided, according to the CDC. The CDC recommends clean water, saline solution, or commercial ophthalmic solutions for washing the eyes.

7. You should establish a network with local emergency personnel, the CDC, laboratories, and state and local health agencies in case of a bioterrorism attack. Such a network would be helpful if a large outbreak occurs.

Appendix B

Sample incident command system

Camden-Clark Memorial Hospital

Emergency Preparedness Management Plan

Note: The following pages are excerpts taken from Camden-Clark Memorial Hospital's incident command system (ICS). This is to be used as a sample only. This is not the ICS in its entirety.

TITLE: Emergency Preparedness Management Plan
FORMULATED BY:
EFFECTIVE DATE:

Purpose:

To provide a plan for the operation of Camden-Clark Memorial Hospital when, due to internal or external events, the normal operation of the hospital is so compromised that its ability to deliver care to patients and/or provide a safe environment is in question or is no longer possible.

Statement:

Camden-Clark Memorial Hospital, in its mission to meet the healthcare needs of our community for a lifetime, considers emergency preparedness a crucial event. The Board of Trustees, medical staff, and administration have established and provide ongoing support for the Emergency Preparedness program as hereby defined.

The purpose of the Emergency Preparedness Management Plan is to provide resources for the continuation of patient care during a variety of emergencies that may disrupt operations at Camden-Clark Memorial Hospital. The plan includes processes designed to provide for the medical and safety needs of patients as a result of an internal or external incident or event.

Scope:

The emergency preparedness program is designed to assure appropriate staff response to a wide variety of emergency situations. The primary emphasis is on short-term management of critical patient care and facility safety during emergency situations. The emergency preparedness plan applies to all staff employed by Camden-Clark Memorial Hospital.

Fundamentals:

- Emergencies will occur. Effective planning reduces the impact of emergencies on the quality of patient care and increases the hospital's ability to continue to provide necessary patient services.
- Many types of emergencies can be identified from past organizational or community experiences. Evaluating past experiences provides a baseline of likely threats in future emergencies. Planning should include responses to these likely situations.
- Planning considers hospital facilities, space, personnel, supplies, communications and other resources needed to provide essential services under less than ideal conditions.

- Planning considers on-duty and off-duty staff and other staff resources when determining what staff is needed to maintain essential services.
- Planning considers conditions that may require modifications of normal patient care routines, including treatment. The conditions may require discontinuation of services, patient transfer, facility evacuation, or discharge of patients.
- Period drills are essential for maintaining staff awareness of emergency procedures and for evaluating the effectiveness of the plan.
- Scheduled drills and actual implementations of the Emergency Preparedness Management Plan are observed, documented, and critiqued to identify opportunities for improvement. Actions taken to address deficiencies are documented and tested during subsequent drills. Summaries of the Emergency Preparedness Management Plan activities are presented to the Safety Committee for review and recommendations.

Goals and objectives:

- Emergency Preparedness Management Plan drills are scheduled four to eight months apart. At least two (2) emergency preparedness drills are conducted each year. No more than one actual implementation will be accepted in lieu of a planned drill each year.
- Implementations are documented and critiqued. Findings are used to identify opportunities to improve the planning process, the Emergency Preparedness Management Plan or a plan scenario, staff training, or the resources available to staff during emergency situations.
- Providing training for all staff required to respond to emergency situations. Training is specific to staff roles and responsibilities. Training includes use of personal protective equipment or other specialized equipment required to be used or operated.
- Identification of key problems, failures, and user errors requiring attention and action.

- Identification of performance improvement standards, collection and analysis of data, and reporting to the Safety Committee.
- Identification of opportunities to improve emergency preparedness performance, planning, response, and staff training.
- Conducting an annual evaluation of the objectives, scope, performance, and effectiveness of the Emergency Preparedness Management Plan and reporting the results to the Safety Committee.

Organization and responsibility:

- The Board of Trustees receives regular reports of the activities of the Emergency Preparedness Management Plan from the Safety Committee. The Board of Trustees reviews the reports and, as appropriate, communicates concerns about identified issues and regulatory compliance. The Board of Trustees provides support to facilitate the ongoing activities of the Emergency Preparedness Management Plan.
- The Chief Executive Officer (CEO) receives regular reports of the current status of the Emergency Preparedness Management Plan through the Safety Committee. The CEO reviews the reports and, as necessary, communicates concerns about key issues and regulatory compliance to the Emergency Preparedness Committee, which, in collaboration with the Safety Committee, is responsible for managing all aspects of the Emergency Preparedness Management Plan. The Emergency Preparedness Committee advises the Safety Committee regarding emergency preparedness issues that may necessitate changes in policies and procedures, orientation or education, or expenditure of funds.
- Department directors and managers are responsible for orienting new personnel to the department and, as appropriate, to the job and task-specific responsibilities for emergency preparedness. Where necessary, the Safety and Security Supervisor provides technical assistance.
- Individual personnel are responsible for learning and following job- and task-specific procedures for emergency response.

Processes of the Emergency Preparedness Management Plan

Program Elements:

- Plans are in place for responses to a variety of emergency and disaster situations that may cause an influx of patients, or compromise the ability of the hospital to provide patient care or a safe environment. These include a mass casualty response plan and plans to respond to weather emergencies such as wind (tornado) or winter weather (ice and snow obstructions to hospital access and staff activity); failures or malfunctions of utility systems (e.g., including water loss or contamination by sewage, loss of electrical power, loss of heating or cooling, etc.); communications failures; and other related procedures.
- The hospital is a member of the county emergency planning council, and meets with the planning council generally on a monthly basis. The hospital participates in plans for emergencies, including medical emergencies and its role in community-wide disasters. On a periodic basis, the county emergency planning council conducts emergency drills, generally including a number of "victims" who are used to test the hospital's mass casualty plan, as well as the local EMS triage and transport plans and other agency plans related to a community-wide emergency. Other agencies, such as the Red Cross, local radio operators, and others are included in the drills. Post drill critiques include the activity of the hospital, as well as other agencies who interface with the hospital during the exercise.
- A variety of emergencies require notification of local, state, or federal agencies in case of emergencies. These include: fire and police agencies; state environmental and labor (safety) agencies; and federal agencies, including OSHA, EPA, and the Coast Guard. Incidents that require such notifications are identified in the Emergency Operations Manual, along with the agency involved and current telephone numbers.

- Staff members are notified when the Emergency Preparedness Management Plan is required by the ICS. Internal staff members are notified by the use of the audible page system and a series of coded announcements. The codes are found on the page attached to the end of this plan. In addition to the audible codes, key staff are paged or telephoned to assure they are aware of the implementation.

Where it is necessary to recall staff or to obtain additional staff to assist with an additional load, the staff members are recalled by use of a telephone tree or cascade system. Each department maintains a current telephone tree, and, as directed by the director or senior person present during the emergency (or by designated staff, if no one is available for that activity), the calling systems are activated to notify additional staff to return to the hospital. Such plans are activated on a periodic basis by the departments to assure currency.

- Where sufficient staff are not available for all roles during an implementation of the plans (such as during a less fully staffed shift), the Incident Command Staff will assure that most critical jobs are filled with available staff and less critical jobs are filled by staff returning to the facility. Lists of key staff roles are available to the disaster incident commanders for their use.
- A number of minor modifications are made during the implementation of various plans. For example, the cafeteria becomes a minor treatment area for a mass-casualty action, and patients are moved to corridors and interior rooms during tornado alerts, and there are similar changes in the normal use of space and facilities in other plans. These space modifications are tested as part of the normal drill exercises, and their use is also evaluated during actual activation of the plan.
- An activation of the hospital for situations that render the facility no longer capable of providing necessary patient care activities. They will be notified as soon as the potential for the need to evacuate is

considered and will be kept updated on an ongoing basis, to begin the process for identification of the availability of space to move the patients. As practical, patients will be moved to sites where their care can be continued and they will be safe.

Plans for non-fire evacuations of the facility include methods to control the movement of patients to the points of debarkation and to move patients safely and with minimum risk in transportation. Non-ambulatory patients will generally move through the main entrance to buses or vans as available. Patients being discharged to their homes and family will move through the Emergency Department entrance.

As is practical, patients being moved to alternate care facilities will be moved with their records (available from their nursing units) and applicable medications.

- Alternate care sites include adjacent hospitals with which reciprocal agreements are maintained. Alternate care sites are selected to assure that patient care will be continued and to provide for patient safety.
- Modifications in patient care include: the discontinuing of elective surgery and other elective procedures; movement of patients to alternate beds within the hospital as deemed appropriate by the incident command staff; implementation of the patient information system (i.e., TriCard System during mass casualty incidents, or incidents where victims come to the facility) to provide a medical record of incoming patients; and implementation and maintenance of a patient log for hospital and public information.
- Alternate sources for utility supplies are defined both in terms of the immediate response of equipment and backup systems and in terms of clinical and patient care activity modifications and reactions to assure patient safety and continued care. In some cases, such as electrical power, backup systems are in place.

Camden-Clark Memorial Hospital

Hospital Policy

TITLE: Activation of Hospital Emergency Preparedness Management Plan
WRITTEN BY: Emergency Preparedness Committee
EFFECTIVE DATE: October 1999
PURPOSE: To provide for the activation of the Emergency Preparedness Management Plan under emergency or potential emergency conditions.

POLICY: In the event of one (1) or more of the following conditions, the Emergency Preparedness Plan may be activated.

- The sudden or expected influx of victims into the Emergency Department that exceeds its capacity to provide patient care in a manner consistent with good patient management.
- An internal event that, because of its nature, disrupts the hospital's ability or has the potential to disrupt the hospital's ability to deliver patient care and/or provide a safe environment.

Examples:

- Fire or smoke event
- Hazardous materials incident
- Utility failure

- An external event that, because of its nature, effects or has the potential to disrupt the hospital's ability to deliver patient care and/or provide a safe environment.

Examples:

- Fire or smoke event
- Hazardous materials incident
- Utility failure
- Severe weather or a potential severe weather event

ACTIVATION: It shall be the responsibility of the activating party to notify the hospital operator, who shall then announce on the hospital paging system that the "Hospital Emergency Plan has been Activated" three (3) times.

Implementation:

- All employees not in their area should immediately return to their respective units.
- Each unit should refer to its EPMP Specific Departmental Guidelines.
- These guidelines, which refer to notification of department personnel and preparation of equipment needed in the event of a disaster, are to be implemented as needed to meet assigned responsibilities determined by the Incident Command System.
- All departments shall continue normal operations unless directed by the Disaster Director and/or the Incident Command System to assume responsibility for specific operations in response to the emergency event.

Camden-Clark Memorial Hospital

Emergency Preparedness Management Plan

Ambulance Service Sector

Responsibility:

Organize and coordinate the operation of the Ambulance Service to provide for its effective operation under the ICS during emergency situations.

IMMEDIATE RESPONSE:

___ Receive appointment from Emergency Department Sector.

___ Obtain information packet and identification vest. Read this job action sheet and review organizational chart.

___ Put on position identification vest.

___ Receive briefing on situation from Emergency Department Sector.

___ Assess available staff and equipment and project needs based on available information.

___ Develop and implement an Action Plan based on the current situation.

___ Initiate staff recall procedure, and initiate requests for additional equipment and ambulances as required.

___ Report operational status and updates on a routine basis to the Emergency Department Sector.

INTERMEDIATE AND LONG-TERM RESPONSE:

___ Project and report ability to deliver critical services and needs under current and/or projected situation for 4, 8, 24, and 48 hours.

___ Monitor effectiveness of Action Plan and modify as necessary for effective operation or to adjust for situation changes.

___ Conduct unit update briefings as necessary.

___ Communicate with Emergency Department Sector as required.

___ Participate in resolving area emergencies.

___ Monitor staff performance and relieve staff for nutrition and rest as required.

___ Assist in the formulation and implementation of plan for return to normal staffing and operation.

___ Assist in the formulation and implementation of plan for retrieval, receipt, and reintegration of patients transferred to other facilities.

Camden-Clark Memorial Hospital

Emergency Preparedness Management Plan

Lead Communicator

Position Assigned To: ______________________________

You Report To: ______________________________

Radio Designation: ______________________________

Emergency Operations Center (EOC) Phone Number:

____

Responsibility:

Maintain current information regarding incident status for the Disaster Director. Assist in the development/operation of the internal/external communication network as needed for effective operation of the EOC. Monitor the need for modification of current communication system and/or assist in the establishment of alternate communication to support assignment. Record events and provide status information to the Disaster Director.

IMMEDIATE RESPONSE:

___ Receive appointment from Disaster Director.

___ Obtain information packet and identification vest. Read this job action sheet and review organizational chart.

___ Put on position identification vest.

___ Receive situation briefing from Disaster Director and/or appropriate Division.

___ Determine needs established by organizational chart and implement necessary contacts and message routing procedures to support position.

___ Transmit and receive information as required to support assignment.

___ Set up event recording forms and equipment and maintain accurate log of events and actions as implemented or received.

___ Coordinate communications with operational EOC Divisions and Wood County Emergency Communications.

INTERMEDIATE AND LONG-TERM RESPONSE:

___ Route communications information and updates as required.

___ Monitor communications system for operational efficiency and ability to fulfill operational needs.

___ Relay special or urgent information to appropriate personnel.

___ Assist in termination and critique of incident.

Camden-Clark Memorial Hospital

Emergency Preparedness Management Plan

Communications Leader

Position Assigned To: ____________________________

You Report To: ____________________________

Radio Designation: ____________________________

EOC Phone Number: ____________________________

Responsibility:

Monitor the status of hospital communications systems and, where necessary, make emergency repairs and/or assist in the establishment of alternate communication systems to supplement, enhance, or replace existing systems.

IMMEDIATE RESPONSE:

___ Receive appointment from Building Services Sector.

___ Obtain information packet and identification vest. Read this job

action sheet and review organizational chart.

___ Put on position identification vest.

___ Receive briefing on situation from Building Services Sector.

___ Access operational status of building communication systems.

___ Develop and implement a priority-based Action Plan based on the current situation.

___ Request additional supplies, equipment, and/or staff as needed to implement Action Plan.

___ Implement staff recall, if required.

___ Report operational status and updates on a routine basis to the Building Services Sector.

___ Report unused staff to Staff Allocation.

INTERMEDIATE AND LONG-TERM RESPONSE:

___ Project and report ability to deliver critical services and needs under current and/or projected situation for 4, 8, 24, and 48 hours.

___ Monitor effectiveness of Action Plan and modify as necessary for effective operation or to adjust for situation changes.

___ Communicate with Building Services Sector as required.

___ Participate in resolving Area emergencies.

___ Monitor staff performance and relieve staff for nutrition and rest as required.

___ Assist in the formulation and implementation of plan for return to normal staffing and operation.

Camden-Clark Memorial Hospital

Emergency Preparedness Management Plan

Crisis Management Sector

Position Assigned To: ______________________________

You Report To: ______________________________

Radio Designation: ______________________________

EOC Phone Number: ______________________________

Responsibility:

Coordinate and provide an integrated information and support system for victims' families/significant others and victims, by designating an appropriate area for their reception, providing information and emotional support and caring for nutritional and physical needs.

IMMEDIATE RESPONSE:

___ Receive appointment from the Public Relations/Welfare Division.

___ Obtain information packet and identification vest. Read this job action sheet and review organizational chart.

___ Put on position identification vest.
___ Receive situation briefing from Public Relations/Welfare Division or others as appropriate.
___ Establish a secure reception area for victims' families/significant others away from the general public, media, EOC, and patient care activities.
___ Assemble needed staff (internal and/or external) to support the functions of this Sector. Contact Staff Allocation Sector for additional staff when appropriate.
___ Brief all staff and detail operational plans and procedure for release of information to families/significant others.
___ Coordinate with the Security Sector to assure the security of the reception/family area.
___ Coordinate with Medical Division to assure the accurate delivery of victim information to family/significant others in an appropriate manner.
___ Coordinate with Public Relations/Welfare to assist individuals requesting information or location of possible victims either at this facility or located at other facilities.
___ Coordinate with Resource Management Division to provide for the physical and nutritional needs of victims' families/significant others.

INTERMEDIATE RESPONSE:
___ Project and report ability to deliver critical services and needs under current and/or projected situation for 4, 8, 24, and 48 hours.
___ Conduct update briefings with staff as required.
___ Communicate with Public Relations/Welfare Division as required.
___ Participate in resolving Sector emergencies.
___ Monitor status of support activities to ensure adequate allocation of resources.
___ Work with area agencies, groups, or resources to support the delivery of both short- and longer-term emotional and physical support.
___ Monitor staff performance and relieve staff for nutrition and rest as required.

Camden-Clark Memorial Hospital

Emergency Preparedness Management Plan

Damage Control Sector

Position Assigned To: ______________________________

You Report To: ______________________________

Radio Designation: ______________________________

EOC Phone Number: ______________________________

Responsibility:

Monitor the physical condition of the facility for the purpose of making decisions about evacuation, relocation, and/or cessation of medical care services. Manage search and rescue operations in the hospital facilities and mitigate damage to minimize the impact on operations and safety.

IMMEDIATE RESPONSE:

___ Receive appointment from the Building Services Sector.

___ Obtain information packet and identification vest. Read this job

action sheet and review organizational chart.

___ Put on position identification vest.

___ Appoint a damage assessment team.

___ Conduct a damage assessment of the facility and report findings to the Building Services Sector.

___ Identify hazards such as unstable structure, non-functional utility services, and other non-functional equipment required for facility operations, and determine the need for victim rescue activities.

___ Organize functional response teams or groups to manage prioritized items as determined above.

___ Supplement existing available staff and/or response groups with available assistance by contacting the Staff Allocation Sector.

___ Conduct re-assessments of the facility at least hourly.

___ Provide regular briefings to the Building Services Sector.

INTERMEDIATE RESPONSE:

___ Project and report ability to deliver critical services and needs under current and/or projected situation for 4, 8, 24, and 48 hours.

___ Arrange for a structural analysis of damaged structures.

___ Photograph damaged areas.

___ Identify areas where immediate salvage should be directed to save critical services and equipment.

___ Arrange for necessary materials and assign staff to salvage duties.

___ Arrange for salvage experts and/or service representatives to conduct long-term recovery operations.

___ Arrange for construction services to stabilize and secure damaged areas.

___ Monitor staff performance and relieve staff for nutrition and rest as required.

Camden-Clark Memorial Hospital

Emergency Preparedness Management Plan

Disaster Director

Position Assigned To: ______________________

Date of Event: __ __ / __ __ / __ __

Type of Event:

____

____

____

Responsibility:

Organize and direct the Emergency Operations Center (EOC). Direct overall hospital operations and coordinate hospital operations with area emergency response agencies. Authorize use of hospital facilities and funds. Authorize evacuation if necessary.

IMMEDIATE RESPONSE:

___ Initiate the Emergency Preparedness Plan by assuming the role of Disaster Director.

___ Read this job action sheet.

___ Put on position identification vest.

___ Establish individuals for the following positions:

  ___ Communicator:

  ____

  ___ Note-Taker:

  ____

___ Appoint Division Leaders appropriate for incident:

  ___ Public Relations/Welfare Division

  ____

  ___ Resource Management Division

  ____

  ___ Medical Division

  ____

  ___ Engineering /Safety Division

  ____

___ Distribute Division Leader packets containing:

- Job Action Sheets for Sector and Group Leaders
- Identification vests for Sector and Group Leaders
- Necessary forms for Sector and Group Leaders

___ Receive initial status reports from Divisions.

___ Determine level of services required and implement appropriate Plan of Action with Division Leaders.

___ Notify Administration of current status and of Action Plan now being undertaken, and establish a briefing cycle to be maintained with Administration.

___ Receive initial damage estimates and determine need for relocation or evacuation.

___ Obtain patient census report and projections for 4, 8, 24, and 48 hours after the incident. Adjust projections as events dictate.

___ Authorize expedited patient assessments and discharges if additional beds are required.
___ Assure contact has been established with outside agencies and off-site staff as dictated by the incident.

INTERMEDIATE RESPONSE:
___ Monitor actions, resources, and needs and authorize modification of the Plan of Action, use of staff, supplies, equipment, and funds to support the Plan of Action as determined by Division operations.
___ Set up briefing schedule with Division Leaders to determine the need for continuation or termination of the EOC and/or EPMP.
___ Approve media releases.
___ Observe staff to determine need for rotation to ensure staff are rested and receive psychological support as needed.
___ Determine food and shelter needs of staff, physicians, volunteers, and dependents. Authorize Support Plan of Action as required.

LONG-TERM RESPONSE:
___ Project and report ability to deliver critical services and needs under current and/or projected situation for 4, 8, 24, and 48 hours.
___ Monitor effectiveness of Plan of Action and modify as necessary for effective operation or to adjust for situation changes.
___ Implement the formulation and implementation of plan for return to normal staffing and operation.
___ Implement the formulation and implementation of plan for retrieval, receipt, and reintegration of patients transferred to other facilities.
___ Initiate a critique of incident with all elements of the Incident Command structure with minutes and accumulation of all documentation from Divisions.
___ Demobilize EOC center.

Camden-Clark Memorial Hospital

Emergency Preparedness Management Plan

Emergency Department Sector

Position Assigned To: ______________________________

You Report To: ______________________________

Radio Designation: ______________________________

EOC Phone Number: ______________________________

Responsibility:

Coordinate the operation of the Emergency Department during emergency conditions. Facilitate the receipt, triage, treatment, transfer to other hospital areas, or their discharge. Facilitate the operation of the Emergency Department and other operational units within the hospital and other services external to the hospital.

IMMEDIATE RESPONSE:

___ Receive appointment from Medical Division.

___ Obtain information packet and identification vest. Read this job action sheet and review organizational chart.
___ Put on position identification vest.
___ Receive briefing on situation from Medical Division.
___ Appoint the following as required. Distribute information packets and identification vests.
  ___ Triage Treatment

  ____

  ___ Immediate Treatment

  ____

  ___ Minor Treatment

  ____

  ___ Delayed Treatment

  ____

___ Situation brief all Treatment Leaders.
___ Develop Action Plan, and request needed resources from Medical Division.
___ Assure propositioned of required supplies.
___ Request additional supplies as dictated by Action Plan.
___ Assess staffing needs and obtain additional staff from Staff Allocation as needed.
___ Initiate staff recall as necessary to meet projected demand.

INTERMEDIATE AND LONG-TERM RESPONSE:
___ Project and report ability to deliver critical services and needs under current and/or projected situation for 2, 4, and 6 hours.
___ Report emergency needs to Medical Division.
___ Request additional projected supply needs to Resource Management Division.
___ Report status of unit frequently to Medical Division.
___ Facilitate the resolution of problems within the Emergency Department Sector.
___ Monitor staff assignments to assure rotation of staff for rest and nutrition.
___ Direct non-utilized personnel to the Staff Allocation Sector.

Camden-Clark Memorial Hospital

Emergency Preparedness Management Plan

Engineering/Safety Division

Position Assigned To: ______________________________

You Report To: ______________________________

Radio Designation: ______________________________

EOC Phone Number: ______________________________

Responsibility:

Maintain the integrity of the physical facility. Maintain safety and security programs to assure staff, patient, and visitor safety. Coordinate the operation of emergency response teams.

IMMEDIATE RESPONSE:

___ Receive appointment from the Disaster Director.

___ Obtain information packet and identification vest. Read this job action sheet and review organizational chart.

___ Put on position identification vest.
___ Appoint Note Taker/Communicator.

____

___ Appoint and brief the following as required. Distribute information packets and identification vests.
  ___ Building Services Sector

  ____

  ___ Security Sector

  ____

___ Activate Chemical Response Team

____

___ Activate Fire Control Team

____

___ Brief Sector Leaders, outline immediate needs, and establish next briefing time.
___ Coordinate damage and security assessments as soon as possible.
___ Initiate emergency actions necessary to obtain or continue a safe operational environment.
___ Brief the Disaster Director on the status of the physical facility and its security.
___ Assign staff or response groups to critical facility operational functions.
___ Provide assistance as required for outside emergency response organizations and/or contractual damage repair operations.
___ Initiate call-back procedure as required.

INTERMEDIATE RESPONSE:
___ Project and report ability to deliver critical services and needs under current and/or projected situation for 4, 8, 24, and 48 hours.
___ Monitor the condition of the facility.
___ Provide continued coordination for emergency and contractual damage control groups.
___ Receive regular briefings from Section Leaders.

___ Provide regular briefings to the Disaster Director.
___ Prepare for evacuation or relocation of medical services as appropriate.
___ Monitor staff performance and relieve staff for nutrition and rest as needed.
___ Monitor actions, resources, and needs and authorize modification of the Plan of Action, use of staff, supplies, equipment, and funds to support the Plan of Action as determined by Division operations.

LONG-TERM RESPONSE:
___ Observe staff to determine need for rotation to ensure staff are rested and receive psychological support as needed.
___ Project and report ability to deliver critical services and needs under current and/or projected situation for 4, 8, 24, and 48 hours.
___ Monitor effectiveness of Plan of Action and modify as necessary for effective operation or to adjust for situation changes.
___ Assist in the formulation and implementation of plan for return to normal staffing and operation.
___ Assist in the formulation and implementation of plan for retrieval, receipt, and reintegration of patients transferred to other facilities.
___ Participate in a critique of incident with all elements of the Incident Command structure upon termination of the emergency.

Camden-Clark Memorial Hospital

Emergency Preparedness Management Plan

Fire Control Team Incident Command

Position Assigned To: ______________________________

You Report To: ______________________________

Radio Designation: ______________________________

EOC Phone Number: ______________________________

Responsibility:

Provide coordination for in-house and external fire control units responding to fire and/or potential fire incidents within the hospital.

IMMEDIATE RESPONSE:

___ Receive activation from Engineering/Safety Division.

___ Obtain information packet and identification vest. Read this job action sheet and review organizational chart.

___ Put on position identification vest.

___ Brief Sector Leaders, outline immediate needs, and establish next briefing time.
___ Coordinate Site Assessment.
___ Initiate emergency actions necessary to obtain a safe operational environment or to minimize the effects of the incident on the ability of the facility to deliver patient care.
___ Brief the Engineering/Safety Division on the status of the fire control operation.
___ Assign staff or response groups on a priority basis.
___ Provide coordination as required with outside emergency response to respond to the fire emergency.

INTERMEDIATE AND LONG-TERM RESPONSE:
___ Project and report ability to deliver critical services and needs under current and/or projected situation for 4, 8, 24, and 48 hours.
___ Provide continued coordination for emergency fire control groups.
___ Receive regular briefings from Section Leaders.
___ Provide regular briefings to the Engineering/Safety Division.
___ Prepare for evacuation or relocation of services as appropriate.
___ Monitor staff performance and relieve staff for nutrition and rest as needed.

Camden-Clark Memorial Hospital

Emergency Preparedness Management Plan

Medical Supply Leader

Position Assigned To: ______________________________

You Report To: ______________________________

Radio Designation: ______________________________

EOC Phone Number: ______________________________

Responsibility:

Acquire, maintain, and distribute required medical supplies to support operational requirements of the facility during an emergency response. Facilitate the resupply of these supplies during the recovery phase of the operation.

IMMEDIATE RESPONSE:

___ Receive appointment from the Supply Sector.

___ Obtain information packet and identification vest. Read this job

action sheet and review organizational chart.

___ Put on position identification vest.

___ Receive situation briefing from Supply Sector.

___ Receive briefing from Supply Sector.

___ Dispatch predesignated supply carts to assigned areas.

___ Conduct an assessment of immediate needs for enhancement of medical supplies throughout the hospital.

___ Coordinate the delivery of essential medical supplies from available stocks, and initiate the acquisition and resupply of all essential medical supplies not in stock or used from available stock.

INTERMEDIATE AND LONG-TERM RESPONSE:

___ Project and report ability to deliver critical services and needs under current and/or projected situation for 4, 8, 24, and 48 hours.

___ Communicate with Supply Sector.

___ Resolve Sector emergencies.

___ Identify needs for replenishment of supplies.

___ Contact suppliers and coordinate the purchase and delivery of supplies to the hospital. Coordinate delivery and/or pickup of materials through the Supply Sector.

___ Assist the Pharmacy Leader in the supply/resupply of drugs and other pharmacy items.

___ Assist the Supply Sector in establishing a long-term recovery plan as required.

Camden-Clark Memorial Hospital

Emergency Preparedness Management Plan

Media Management Sector

Position Assigned To: ______________________________

You Report To: ______________________________

Radio Designation: ______________________________

EOC Phone Number: ______________________________

Responsibility:

Provide for the coordinated flow of information to the news media during emergency events by designating an appropriate area for the reception of news media, and arranging for the routine release of information to the news media by hospital staff or other appropriate individuals.

IMMEDIATE RESPONSE:

___ Receive appointment from the Public Relations/Welfare Division.
___ Obtain information packet and identification vest. Read this job

action sheet and review organizational chart.
___ Put on position identification vest.
___ Receive situation briefing from Public Relations/Welfare Division or others as appropriate.
___ Establish media relations center away from the EOC and patient care activities.
___ Assemble needed support staff and detail operational guidelines and news release restrictions.
___ Issue initial information report to the news media.

INTERMEDIATE AND LONG-TERM RESPONSE:
___ Project and report ability to deliver critical services and needs under current and/or projected situation for 4, 8, 24, and 48 hours.
___ Conduct update briefings with news media.
___ Communicate with Public Relations/Welfare Division as required.
___ Issue periodic news releases approved by the Disaster Director.
___ Participate in resolving Sector emergencies.
___ Determine requests for assistance to be made to the public through the media.
___ Continue media briefings.
___ Monitor status of support activities to ensure adequate allocation of resources.
___ Work with area agencies to reduce the number of individuals requiring basic support services at the hospital.
___ Monitor staff performance and relieve staff for nutrition and rest as required.

Camden-Clark Memorial Hospital

Emergency Preparedness Management Plan

Respiratory Care Unit Leader

Position Assigned To: ______________________________

You Report To: ______________________________

Radio Designation: ______________________________

EOC Phone Number: ______________________________

Responsibility:

Provide respiratory care services and staff sufficient to meet the needs of victims of emergency incidents and the current patient load.

IMMEDIATE RESPONSE:

___ Receive appointment from Supportive Sector.

___ Obtain information packet and identification vest. Read this job action sheet and review organizational chart.

___ Put on position identification vest.

___ Receive briefing from Supportive Sector Leader.
___ Evaluate current service delivery capability and supplies.
___ Provide technicians and portable equipment to Immediate and Delayed treatment areas as required.
___ Initiate staff call-back as required.

INTERMEDIATE AND LONG-TERM RESPONSE:
___ Project and report ability to deliver critical services and needs under current and/or projected situation for 4, 8, 24, and 48 hours.
___ Monitor supply levels and coordinate acquisition and delivery of supplies with Supply Sector.
___ Report unassigned Respiratory staff to Staff Allocation Sector available for reallocation.
___ Monitor staff duty hours and rotate staff for rest and nutrition.
___ Monitor and report to the Support Sector any modifications in ability to deliver required services.

Camden-Clark Memorial Hospital

Emergency Preparedness Management Plan

Security Sector

Position Assigned To: ______________________________

You Report To: ______________________________

Radio Designation: ______________________________

EOC Phone Number: ______________________________

Responsibility:

Monitor the safety and security conditions in the buildings and on the campus. Take action to restore safe and secure conditions.

IMMEDIATE RESPONSE:

___ Receive appointment from the Engineering/Safety Division Leader.

___ Obtain information packet and identification vest. Read this job action sheet and review organizational chart.

___ Put on position identification vest.

___ Appoint a safety and security assessment team.
___ Conduct an assessment of the facility and report findings to the Engineering/Safety Division.
___ Identify needs for the control of safety and/or security throughout the organization.
___ Initiate call-back procedure as required.
___ Contact the Staff Allocation Sector to obtain staff to manage safety or security as required to supplement existing staff.
___ Remove unauthorized personnel from restricted areas.
___ Assist all Sector and Unit Leaders to secure space and prepare it for use.
___ Conduct reassessments of the facility at least hourly.
___ Provide regular briefings to the Engineering/Safety Division.

INTERMEDIATE AND LONG-TERM RESPONSE:
___ Project and report ability to deliver critical services and needs under current and/or projected situation for 4, 8, 24, and 48 hours.
___ Immediately notify the Engineering/Safety Division of threats to safety and/or security.
___ Initiate contact with law enforcement to coordinate security activities.
___ Assign staff to transport critical medical and/or operational supplies.
___ Assist in screening, credentialing, and providing identification to outside and volunteer responders.
___ Provide regular briefings for the Engineering/Safety Division.
___ Take action to resolve immediate safety and/or security threats.
___ Monitor staff performance and relieve staff for nutrition and rest as needed.

Appendix C

Critical biological and chemical agents

Below you will find the Centers for Disease Control and Prevention's (CDC) list of category A and B agents.

Biological agents—Category A

The United States public health system and primary healthcare providers must be prepared to address varied biological agents, including pathogens that are rarely seen in the United States.

High-priority agents include organisms that pose a risk to national security because they

- can be easily disseminated or transmitted person-to-person
- cause high mortality, with potential for major public health impact
- might cause public panic and social disruption
- require special action for public health preparedness

Category A agents include the following:

- Variola major (smallpox)
- Bacillus anthracis (anthrax)

- Yersinia pestis (plague)
- Clostridium botulinum toxin (botulism)
- Francisella tularensis (tularaemia)
- Filoviruses
  - Ebola hemorrhagic fever
  - Marburg hemorrhagic fever
- Arenaviruses
  - Lassa (Lassa fever)
  - Junin (Argentine hemorrhagic fever)

Category B

Second highest priority agents include those that

- are moderately easy to disseminate
- cause moderate morbidity and low mortality
- require specific enhancements of the CDC's diagnostic capacity and enhanced disease surveillance

Category B agents include the following:

- Coxiella burnetti (Q fever)
- Brucella species (brucellosis)
- Burkholderia mallei (glanders)
- Alphaviruses
  - Venezuelan encephalomyelitis
  - Eastern and western equine encephalomyelitis
- Ricin toxin from Ricinus communis (castor beans)
- Epsilon toxin of Clostridium perfringens
- Staphylococcus enterotoxin B

A subset of List B agents include pathogens that are food- or waterborne. These pathogens include, but are not limited to, the following:

- Salmonella species
- Shigella dysenteriae
- Escherichia coli O 157:H7

- Vibrio cholerae
- Cryptosporidium parvum

Chemical agents

Chemical agents that might be used by terrorists range from warfare agents to toxic chemicals commonly used in industry. Criteria for determining priority chemical agents include

- chemical agents already known to be used as weaponry
- availability of chemical agents to potential terrorists
- chemical agents likely to cause major morbidity or mortality
- potential of agents for causing public panic and social disruption
- agents that require special action for public health preparedness

Categories of chemical agents include the following:

- Nerve agents
- Blood agents
- Blister agents
- Heavy metals
- Volatile toxins
- Pulmonary agents
- Incapacitating agents
- Pesticides, persistent and nonpersistent
- Dioxins, furans, and polychlorinated biphenyls
- Explosive nitro compounds and oxidizers
- Flammable industrial gases, liquids, and solids
- Corrosive industrial acids and bases

Appendix D

What to do if you receive an anthrax threat

The U.S. Postal Service offers these suggestions on what to do if you receive an anthrax threat in the mail. We include them as an aid to protect your facility from the threat of bioterrorism.

How likely is it that someone would receive a harmful biological or chemical substance in the mail?
The Postal Service delivers approximately 208 billion pieces of mail per year. As of October 16, 2001, there have been only two confirmed incidents of anthrax bacteria being sent through the mail.

What should I do if I receive an anthrax threat by mail?

1. Do not handle the piece of mail or package suspected of contamination.
2. Notify your supervisor, who will immediately contact the Inspection Service, local police, safety officer, or designated person.
3. Make sure that damaged or suspicious packages are isolated and the immediate area cordoned off.

4. Ensure that all persons who have touched the piece of mail wash their hands with soap and water.
5. List all persons who have touched the letter/envelope. Include contact information.
6. Provide the list to the Inspection Service.
7. Place all items worn when in contact with the suspected piece of mail in plastic bags, keep them in the place where you change your clothes, and have them available for law enforcement agents.
8. As soon as possible, shower with soap and water.
9. If prescribed medication by medical personnel, take it until otherwise instructed or until it runs out.
10. The Inspectors will assess the threat situation and coordinate with the FBI.
11. Designated officials will notify local, county, and state health departments.
12. Designated officials will notify the state emergency manager.
13. Notify the Center for Disease Control Emergency Response at 770/488-7100 for answers to any questions.

What constitutes a suspicious letter or parcel?
Some typical characteristics that ought to trigger suspicion include letters or parcels that

- have any powdery substance on the outside
- are unexpected or from someone unfamiliar to you
- are addressed to someone no longer with your organization or are otherwise outdated
- have no return address, or have one that can't be verified as legitimate
- are of unusual weight, given their size, or are lopsided or oddly shaped
- have an unusual amount of tape on them
- are marked with restrictive endorsements, such as "Personal" or "Confidential"
- have strange odors or stains

- show a city or state in the postmark that doesn't match the return address

What should I do if I've received a suspicious letter or parcel in the mail?

- Do not try to open the piece of mail
- Isolate the piece of mail
- Evacuate the immediate area
- Call a Postal Inspector to report that you've received a parcel in the mail that may contain biological or chemical substances

Appendix E

Anthrax and small pox fact sheet

- Anthrax is an acute infectious disease caused by the spore-forming bacterium Bacillus anthracis. Anthrax most commonly occurs in hoofed mammals and can also infect humans.

- Symptoms of the disease vary depending on how the disease was contracted, but usually occur within seven days after exposure. The serious forms of human anthrax are inhalation anthrax, cutaneous anthrax, and intestinal anthrax.

- Initial symptoms of inhalation anthrax may resemble a common cold. After several days, the symptoms may progress to severe breathing problems and shock. Inhalation anthrax is often fatal.

- Cutaneous anthrax occurs after direct contact with infectious spores. It is commonly seen in the form of itchy lesions on the head, forearms, or hands. It is usually not fatal if treated with antibiotics.

- The intestinal disease form of anthrax may follow the consumption of contaminated food and is characterized by an acute inflammation of the intestinal tract. Initial signs of nausea, loss of appetite, vomiting, and fever are followed by abdominal pain, vomiting of blood, and severe diarrhea.

- Direct, person-to-person spread of anthrax is extremely unlikely, if it occurs at all. Therefore, there is no need to immunize or treat those who come in contact with persons ill with anthrax, such as family, friends, or coworkers, unless they were also exposed to the same source of infection.

- In persons exposed to anthrax, infection can be prevented with antibiotic treatment.

- Early antibiotic treatment of anthrax is essential—any delay lessens the chances for survival. Anthrax usually is susceptible to penicillin, doxycycline, and fluoroquinolones.

- An anthrax vaccine can also prevent infection. Vaccination against anthrax is not recommended for the general public to prevent the disease and, in any event, is not available.

Smallpox fact sheet

- Smallpox was eliminated from the world in 1977.

- Smallpox is caused by the variola virus. The incubation period is about 12 days (the range is seven to 17 days) following exposure. Initial symptoms include high fever, fatigue, and head- and backaches. A characteristic rash, most prominent on the face, arms, and legs, follows in 2 - 3 days. The rash starts with flat, red lesions that evolve at the same rate. Lesions become pus-filled and begin to crust early in the second week. Scabs develop and then fall off after about 3 - 4 weeks. The majority of patients with smallpox recover, but death occurs in up to 30% of cases.

- Smallpox is spread from one person to another by infected saliva droplets that expose a susceptible person who has face-to-face contact with the ill person. Persons with smallpox are most infectious during the first week of illness because that is when the largest amount of virus is present in saliva. However, some risk of transmission lasts until all scabs have fallen off.

- Routine vaccination against smallpox ended in 1972. The level of immunity, if any, among persons who were vaccinated before 1972 is uncertain; therefore, these persons are assumed to be susceptible.

- Vaccination against smallpox is not recommended to prevent the disease in the general public and, therefore, is not available.

- In people exposed to smallpox, the vaccine can lessen the severity of or even prevent the illness if given within four days after exposure. The vaccine against smallpox contains another live virus called vaccinia. The vaccine does not contain the smallpox virus.

- The United States currently has an emergency supply of the smallpox vaccine.

- There is no proven treatment for smallpox, but research to evaluate new antiviral agents is ongoing. Patients with smallpox can benefit from supportive therapy (intravenous fluids, medicine to control fever or pain, etc.) and antibiotics for any secondary bacterial infections that occur.

Source: Centers for Disease Control and Prevention.

Appendix F

Think about these questions for your fire drills

When conducting fire drills, Children's Medical Center of Dallas, TX, evaluates the following items:

- Is the overhead code red page audible?
- Do all staff members return to their department when a code red is announced?
- Are all patient room doors closed?
- Do staff members know evacuation procedures?
- Are personnel prepared to evacuate horizontally?
- Do employees know the locations of horizontal smoke compartments?
- Do workers know where the emergency exits are?
- Do workers know the locations of portable fire extinguishers?
- Do the appropriate staff members bring extinguishers to the room of drill origin?
- Do employees know how to operate extinguishers?
- Do employees remove patients from the area of fire origin?
- Do employees pull the fire alarm?
- Do employees shut the door to the room of fire origin?

Appendix G

A dozen tips for better fire/evacuation drills

1. Your facility should have a site identified to which you can transfer residents safely.

2. Minimize warning your staff in advance when you conduct a fire/evacuation drill to make it more life-like.

3. It is always a good idea to check with your local or state public safety regulators for minimum requirements on frequency of drills. To cover several possible scenarios, you should conduct the drill at different times of day and different days of the week. Also, it's important that all staff members and residents take part in these drills, so they know their responsibilities during a fire or emergency.

4. During the drill, alert staff members of what the drill simulates. Is there a fire, earthquake, or gas leak? Is it a blaze in a wastebasket or is a computer on fire? Is there smoke in the corridor?

5. Many employees are hesitant to set off a fire alarm, even in an emergency. Have a disconnected alarm station that they can practice

pulling. The same concept goes for fire extinguishers.

6. Keep an updated roster of the location of your residents and their medications. Make sure someone is in charge of the roster and regularly updating it. During the drill, go through the steps of checking the whereabouts of all residents and staff members.

7. An assigned staff member should take the emergency contact list of residents' family members when exiting the building.

8. Drills should also include quizzing staff members on the locations of fire extinguishers, evacuation destinations, fire alarm pull stations, and other safety features.

9. Have a sufficient number of trained observers to verify that all areas of the building respond properly to a drill, not just those near the simulated fire.

10. Your plan should indicate who is responsible for calling the fire department. Before the drill, check with the fire department to find out whether they will participate in the drill. Then, during the drill, the assigned staff member should be responsible for making the call.

11. Make sure that your staff members perform the entire drill. The drill is not over until everyone is in a safe area, such as a designated smoke compartment or out of the building. You can't just hope that in a real emergency your staff will know what to do if they haven't finished the entire drill.

12. After the drill, evaluate your staff's performance. It is helpful to have evaluation forms on which to summarize problems and offer corrective actions, and that also serve as documentation for authorities and surveyors. Test every part of the plan. Find out how the drill went from the beginning to the end.

Appendix H

Hazard prevention control

The following are some suggestions on beefing up hospital security from Fredrick Roll, executive vice president of Healthcare Security Services in Denver, CO:

1. Install and maintain alarm systems and other security devices, panic buttons, hand-held radios, etc., where risk is apparent.

2. Provide metal detectors where appropriate.

3. Use continuous closed-circuit video in high-risk areas.

4. Enclose nursing stations, install deep service counters or bullet-resistant/shatter-proof glass in reception areas, triage, admitting, or client service rooms.

5. Provide employees with a "safe room" for emergencies.

6. Provide two exits for patient care and counseling rooms.

7. Prohibit employees from working alone in emergency areas or walk-in clinics, particularly at night.

8. Provide staff members with security escorts to parking areas at night; make parking areas visible, well lit, and safely accessible to the building.

9. Designate a contact person to be informed of workers' whereabouts throughout the day.

10. Encourage employees to avoid threatening situations.

11. Develop policies and procedures covering home healthcare providers.

12. Enforce visiting hours and procedures.

13. A trained response team should be in place to respond to emergencies.

14. Administrative and work practice controls should state clearly to patients, clients, and employees that violence is not permitted and will not be tolerated.

Appendix I

Check your facility for winter life safety hazards

This checklist contains items culled from various *Healthcare Life Safety Compliance (HLSC)* stories about winter hazards. Answering "no" to any of the questions indicates the possibility of a winter hazard. We hope this list helps you think about various risks associated with cold weather.

We provide a suggested code or regulatory reference for each question, such as from the *Life Safety Code (LSC)* or the environment of care (EC) standards. The items are not all-inclusive, and facilities may have site-specific problems they need to address.

Walkway and entrance concerns

Have walkways, entrances, doors, and sidewalks been cleared of snow and ice? (*Reference:* Statement of Conditions, *part* 3A, *question* 5M)

Have other means of egress to public ways been cleared of snow and ice? (*Reference:* 1997 LSC, *section* 5-7)

Are indoor walk-off mats at entrances long enough to keep floors dry? *(Reference: EC.1.1)*

Is the illumination of the exterior portions in the means of egress adjusted for winter darkness hours? *(Reference: 1997* LSC, *paragraph* 5-8.1.3)

Roof concerns

Can people on the roof get locked out? *(Reference: EC.1.1)*

Are rooftops cleared of ice and snow when necessary? *(Reference: EC.1.1)*

If your facility has a helicopter pad, does it have adequate freeze protection? *(Reference: NFPA 418,* Heliports, *section* 3-6.4.3)

Pipe and connection concerns

Are fire hydrants, fire department connections, and post indicator valves clear of ice and snow? *(Reference: NFPA 25,* Inspection, Testing, and Maintenance of Water-Based Fire Protection Systems, *paragraphs 4-4.3.2 and 11-6)*

Are fire suppression system pipes protected against possible freezing conditions? *(Reference: NFPA 25, section* 2-2.5)

Are "dry" system pipes free of moisture and freezing? *(Reference: NFPA 13,* Installation of Sprinkler Systems, *section* 4-2.5)

Do "wet" system pipes have the proper antifreeze mixture, if necessary? *(Reference: NFPA 13, section* 4-5)

Is there extra moisture in your fire hydrants or are your hydrants frozen? *(Reference: NFPA 25, paragraph* 4-4.3.2)

Are fire department connections protected against possible freezing conditions? *(Reference: NFPA 13, paragraph 5-15.2.1)*

Miscellaneous concerns

Do you have an emergency preparedness plan in place in case temperatures or bad weather knock down one or more utilities? *(Reference: EC.1.4)*

Are your portable fire extinguishers appropriate to use in freezing conditions? *(Reference: NFPA 10,* Portable Fire Extinguishers, *section C-3.2 of Appendix C)*

Is your emergency generator fuel source reliable (will the fuel gel in extreme temperatures)? *(Reference: NFPA 110,* Emergency and Standby Power Systems, *section 5-9.8)*

Is the generator room temperature and/or engine water jacket within acceptable guidelines? *(Reference: NFPA* Health Care Facilities Handbook, *paragraph 3-4.1.1.9)*

Site-specific concerns

Other concern:____
(Reference:____)

Other concern:____
(Reference:____)

Other concern:____
(Reference:____)

Appendix J

Helpful Web sites

The following is a list of Web sites where additional disaster- and safety-related information can be found.

The Centers for Disease Control and Prevention
www.cdc.gov

The Federal Emergency Management Agency
www.fema.gov

The Food and Drug Administration
www.fda.gov

Healthsafetyinfo.com—our site of important health safety tips and news
www.healthsafetyinfo.com

Johns Hopkins Hospital Safety Manual
www.jhu.edu/~safety/manuals/sfman850.txt

The Joint Commission on Accreditation of Healthcare Organizations
www.jcaho.org

MSDSSearch
www.msdssearch.com

The National Fire Protection Association
www.nfpa.org

The National Institute of Occupational Safety and Health
www.cdc.gov/niosh

The Occupational Safety and Health Administration
www.osha.gov

The following is a list of Web sites where you can find information on infectious diseases, bioterrorism, food-borne diseases, immunization, and trade associations. This list comes from the May 2000 report of the Association of State and Territorial Directors of Health Promotion and Public Health Education (ASTDHPPHE) Model Emergency Response Communications Plan for Infectious Disease, Outbreaks, and Bioterrorist Events.

General

- Centers for Disease Control and Prevention (CDC), National Center for Infectious Diseases
  www.cdc.gov/ncidod
  Contains information about nearly 100 different diseases, as well as downloadable fact sheets on many of the diseases and images of the infectious agents.
- National Institutes of Health (NIH), National Institute of Allergies and Infectious Diseases
  www.niaid.nih.gov
  This site offers news releases as well as information on Division of Microbiology and Infectious Diseases research activities.

Bioterrorism

- CDC Bioterrorism Preparedness & Response Network
  www.bt.cdc.gov
  This site provides information about chemical and biological agents, press releases, training, contacts, and other information dealing with the public health aspects of bioterrorism preparedness and response.

- Federal Bureau of Investigation (FBI)
  www.fbi.gov
  Provides links to FBI field offices and contains copies of FBI press releases, as well as information on major ongoing investigations.

- Soldier Biological and Chemical Command
  www.sbccom.army.mil
  A Department of Defense site addressing chemical and biological warfare agent classifications, etiologies, and recommendations for response.

- U.S. Army Medical Research Institute for Infectious Diseases
  www.usamriid.army.mil

Data

- Morbidity and Mortality Weekly Report (MMWR)
  www.cdc.gov/mmwr
  Provides information on disease trends, access to MMWR publications from 1992 to the present, and hot links to all state health departments and other sites of interest.

- National Center for Health Statistics
  www.cdc.gov/nchs/
  Provides data about a number of infectious diseases. Also provides a search function, tabulated state data, and information and/or links

to a number of federally supported surveys and data collection systems.

Emergency management of infectious disease outbreaks

- Federal Emergency Management Agency
  www.fema.gov
  Provides extensive information on emergency management of all types of disasters, including large-scale infectious outbreaks and bioterrorist incidents.

- National Domestic Preparedness Office
  www.ndpo.gov
  The National Domestic Preparedness Office coordinates all federal efforts to assist state and local first responders with planning, training, and equipment to respond to a conventional or non-conventional weapon of mass destruction incident.

- National Emergency Management Association, NEMA
  www.nemaweb.org
  This site contains NEMA policy statements, links to state emergency management contacts, and emergency management information and assistance resources for state officials.

Foodborne disease

- CDC FoodNet
  www.cdc.gov/ncidod/dbmd/foodnet
  The Web site for the CDC Foodborne Diseases Active Surveillance Network (FoodNet), FoodNet is a collaborative project among CDC, several state and local Emerging Infectious Program sites, the U.S. Department of Agriculture, and the U.S. Food and Drug Administration.

- U.S. Department of Agriculture (USDA)
  www.usda.gov
  You can access resources for food safety educators, consumer information (including a listing of product recalls), news releases, and USDA food safety publications.

- U.S. Food and Drug Administration (FDA)
  www.fda.gov
  The U.S. FDA provides general information on food safety, information about the National Food Safety Institute, links to other sites, and information for kids and educators.

Immunizations

- CDC Immunizations Hotline
  Hotline numbers are 1-800-232-2522 (English) and 1-800-232-0233 (Spanish).

- National Coalition for Adult Immunization
  www.nfid.org/ncai
  From this site, you can download adult and adolescent immunization schedules, identify state and local agencies with whom you might collaborate on adult immunization programs, and order educational materials.

- National Immunization Program
  www.cdc.gov/NIP/
  Here you will find current recommended immunization schedules for children and adults and be able to access additional NIP reference materials and publications.

- Vaccines for Children Program (VFC)
  www.cdc.gov/NIP/vfc
  This site lists information about the VFC program and the Advisory Committee on Immunization Practices.

Professional associations

- Association for Professionals in Infection Control and Epidemiology
  www.apic.org
  Contains information on infectious diseases and hospital settings, including a "Bioterrorism Readiness Plan." The plan provides a general overview of what hospitals and other healthcare entities need to consider when developing emergency response procedures for bioterrorism incidents.

- Council of State and Territorial Epidemiologists
  www.cste.org
  The site offers a list of diseases and conditions that healthcare providers and laboratories must report in each state.

- National Emergency Management Association (NEMA), *www.nemaweb.org*
  The NEMA site has links to state emergency management contacts, and emergency management information and assistance resources for state officials.